Breast Cancer and You

Bettering the Odds

With best wishes for health and happiness

Martha Grigg

How to Join the Increasing Number of Women Who Survive, Whole and Well

Martha Grigg
A Breast Cancer Survivor

BRANDEN PUBLISHING COMPANY
Boston

Library of Congress Cataloging-in-Publication Data

Grigg, Martha L.
　　Breast cancer and you : bettering the odds : how to
join the increasing number of women who survive-- whole
and well / by Martha L. Grigg.
　　　　　p. cm.
　　Includes bibliographical references and index.
　　ISBN 0-8283-2010-1 (trade paper)
　　1. Breast--Cancer--Popular works.
　　I. Title.
　　RC280.B8G73 1955
　　616.99'449--dc20　　　　　　　　　　　　95-20816
　　　　　　　　　　　　　　　　　　　　　　　　　CIP

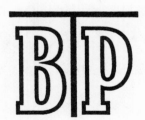

BRANDEN PUBLISHING COMPANY, Inc.
17 Station Street
Box 843 Brookline Village
Boston, MA 02147

To Bill

for his love and support as husband, lover and friend

and for his tremendous help with this book

The intention of this book is to give the reader an overview of what breast cancer is and possible options for treatment of the disease. The information is as accurate as the author could make it. Patients and their families and friends should not, however, use this book or the information in it as substitutes for diagnosis and treatment by health care professionals.

ACKNOWLEDGEMENTS

For their medical and/or editorial help and support, many thanks to: Roberta Ankenbrandt, Phyllis Beardsley; James D'Angelo, M.D.; Ruth Dupree, P.T.; Mary K. Fisher; Eileen Guzikowski; Karen Hall; Chris Hejtmancik, R.N. B.S.N.; Virginia Hutchinson; Emilio Ramos, M.D., Associate Professor of Medicine, the University of Maryland School of Medicine; Jane Ramos, R.N. B.A.N.; and Thomas J. Sanzaro, M.D.

A special thank-you to my dear friend Nancy Marsh for her guidance and time spent in preparing this manuscript. And thanks to Pat Grigsby for her technical expertise.

And to my wonderful family and friends -- I couldn't have done it without you!

And cheers to my fellow "bosom buddies" for their sharing and caring: Alice, Barbara, Bonnie, Carolyn, Dolores, Doris, Dorothy, Eileen, Jane, Janet, Janie, Joni, Judy, Marty, Mary K., Nancy, and Phyllis.

In loving memory of three who didn't make it: Amelia Manning, April McLearn, Martha Wold Olson Ward.

Cover design by Karen Hall
Cover photo by Bill Grigg

TABLE OF CONTENTS

1. BREAST CANCER!

Perhaps it started with a lump that you found yourself. It might have been the first one you ever discovered or perhaps this one felt "different." Or maybe it began with an agonizing moment when your doctor's examining fingers suddenly stopped in their probe of your breast and went over the same area again, this time with a certain urgency. The doctor didn't say anything, except perhaps something about "palpable mass," but there was something different about his or her eyes.

"What's the matter?" you might have gotten up the courage to ask.

And the doctor replied, "We'll talk about it in my office after you're dressed."

And later, "It's probably nothing, but we need to do some more tests."

Or even before there was a lump big enough to feel, if you're "lucky," you have your mammogram and suddenly you feel a difference in the technician's attitude after she returns from making sure the x-rays have come out. More mammograms are done.

Other times, there is a surprise phone call: The doctor wants to see you, and you realize you haven't heard the results of your mammogram.

Or, when you meet your doctor for an analysis of your physical, he or she says, "There seems to be something suspicious on your mammogram. It is probably a cyst, but we'll need to do a needle aspiration." (Whatever that is, you wonder to yourself.) Or perhaps you are told there were microcalcifications on your mammogram and the doctor explains that these sometimes gather around cancer cells.

"I will make an appointment for you to see a surgeon. He may recommend a biopsy."

Perhaps you hear such phrases as:

"Hope for the best but expect the worst."

"It's probably only a fibroadenoma."

"This has to come out right away."

Or you wake up from the biopsy and through a blur of anesthesia you see the surgeon's green outfit and then his or her face. "I'm sorry, but we did find some cancer."

About 180,000 women a year in the United States -- or about one in eight over their lifetime -- hear this bad news, but that doesn't make it easier when it happens to you.

EMOTIONS AND BREAST CANCER

Breast cancer. The words are terrifying. It's a nightmare we all dread.

"Stark terror," was the answer my friend Eileen Guzi-kowski gave me when I asked her to describe her emotions when the first diagnosis came in.

Then there is anger: "Why me? Why was I singled out for this?"

Or guilt: "If I'd had a better diet, had drunk less alcohol, had had children earlier...."

There is the feeling that you have something akin to leprosy, and the fear that you will be rejected by your husband, lover, children, friends.

And there is grief. Betty Rollin, who along with Rose Kushner, was one of the pioneers in changing attitudes towards alternative breast cancer treatments, titled one of her books, *First, You Cry.*

There is the very real fear that you will die. Not quickly, but after a painful, lingering illness filled with drastic chemotherapy. Actor Pierce Brosnan, a fierce advocate for more research after his wife lost her fight with ovarian cancer, put it this way: "Cancer is a six-letter word that knows no boundaries."[1]

And how about anxiety for your home, your family, your job? How about disfigurement? Hair loss?

What about your body? Will you ever feel attractive again after surgery, radiation, chemotherapy? What about sex, your looks, hormonal changes in your body?

You may also feel a total loss of control over your life. Time may seem to pass so quickly that you feel swept overboard with people all around you telling you what to do. Or time may creep, especially when you are waiting for the results of tests or surgery or are undergoing chemotherapy.

You may want to deny that all this is happening to you and become passive when you should be finding out about your disease and making decisions yourself.

Unless you are a "super woman," you will experience some or all of these emotions. At the same time, you will be undergoing various procedures to determine the extent of your cancer. And you will be expected to make some decisions about your treatment.

How can you be expected to cope? How can you make decisions that will influence the rest of your life? To make decisions that may save your life? Knowing you have cancer, isn't it hard enough just to get up in the morning and face the world?

The first thing you need to do is to come to terms with your emotions. You can expect a roller coaster of feelings, depending on what the doctors say, what the diagnostic tests show, and what your options turn out to be.

Since you are reading this book, however, it is obvious that you are not a quitter. You want to find out more. And you are ready to fight.

Of course your emotions are in turmoil. *Of course* you are scared shitless, and more importantly, witless. *Of course* you burst into tears in your doctor's office, at home over dinner, or while talking to a relative or friend on the phone.

This behavior is normal. Every emotion at this time is normal.

Everything else in your life will be second to your disease for a time. You need to plan and to try to make this traumatic event an opportunity. You'll probably do some things differently once this is behind you. You may even lose some friends, but you will also make new ones.

Eileen describes the whole ordeal of breast cancer as a time of "catastrophic loss." But while it is perfectly normal to be a traumatized basket case part of the time, you must also understand that you have rational decisions to make, and soon. For those decisions, knowledge is essential. You need to keep your wits sufficiently to be able to learn everything possible about your breast cancer, your options, and the pros and cons of the various treatments available.

You must stay in control of your life as much as possible. There are some things, of course, that are out of your power. Once the decision about the course of your treatment is made, you cannot control the major effects of surgery, radiation, or chemotherapy.

WHY BREAST CANCER IS SO DANGEROUS

You are dealing with a very dangerous enemy. Most breast cancer is insidious, like a guerrilla army, moving and adapting. Breast cancer cells can travel through the lymph system, starting with the lymph nodes under your arm or with those under your chest wall, or they can go through the blood stream. The army may strike back in the same area or it may move on to other parts of the body, mainly the liver, bones, lungs and brain, or to the skin or even to the pericardial sac that surrounds the heart. These cells can then adapt themselves to the new location and grow there.

The spread can be fast or slow. Breast cancer cells can lie dormant for many years before beginning to grow. Or more aggressive forms can spread with terrifying speed.

The unpredictability and adaptability of breast cancer cells are among the reasons that doctors often feel aggressive measures must be taken to get rid of every single cell that might be left behind after surgery. The options that doctors have to offer seem amazingly primitive: For the most part they can either cut (surgery), burn (radiation), or poison (chemotherapy) the breast cancer cells.

More treatments are being developed all the time, however, and some newer drugs such as tamoxifen have fewer serious side effects. The Pharmaceutical Manufacturers Association recently reported 37 medicines currently being clinically tested to fight breast cancer.[2]

SOME POSITIVES

There is other good news. Most women *do* benefit from their treatments for early breast cancers.

"We're no longer talking about five-year survival rates," says Dr. Stanley A. Schwartz, a prominent oncologist (a specialist in treating cancer) in the Washington, D.C. area. "We're looking at 10 and 15 years and beyond."

Rejoice, at least a little, because in 1992, comprehensive reviews of treatment studies worldwide provided you and your doctor with the some good "insider" bets on the best treatments. This overview proved conclusively that chemotherapy and/or the hormonal drug tamoxifen could prolong life as well as cut the possibility of recurrence.[3]

And be glad you didn't get breast cancer in 1950, 1960, 1970 or even 1980, when most women automatically had a mastectomy, and "breast conservation" was regarded with raised eyebrows in much of the medical community. Not only that, but a woman had to sign away her breast in consenting to

Breast Cancer Death Rates

These figures, released in January 1995,
showed breast cancer rates declining for white women.

Breast Cancer Trends Among U.S. Women		
	Percent change in mortality rate over the indicated period	
Age range (White women)	1989-92	1987-92
30-39	-8.7	-17.8
40-49	-8.1	
50-59	-9.3	
60-69	-4.8	
70-79	-3.4	
80 and above	+1.0	
White women (all ages)	-5.5	
Black women (all ages)	+2.6	
All women	-4.7	

Journal of the National Cancer Institute

have a biopsy! Can you imagine the terror involved in not knowing whether you'd wake up with or without a breast?

When I was first married, in the 1970s, I had my own personal traumatic experience with this type of treatment. I had to have a lump biopsied, and before the procedure could be done, I had to give permission for the surgeon to remove my breast immediately if a quickie test (frozen section) showed cancer!

As a matter of fact, I had to sign away *both* breasts because there had been a paperwork mixup. And then the paperwork didn't get fixed. In the operating room, the anesthesiologist wanted to hook up the wrong arm. As the anesthesia started to take hold, I drunkenly asked my surgeon, "Doctor, are you sure you know where this lump is?"

I can laugh now, because I came out fine. The tissue was benign, but that didn't erase the two weeks of severe anxiety that preceded the operation.

Now women don't have to go through the trauma of not knowing if they will wake up with or without a breast. Biopsies themselves are becoming more refined and the tissue removed can provide more information about the kind of cancer found. And, a new computerized system for analyzing cells taken out during a "needle" biopsy shows promise and may eventually even eliminate the need for lymph node surgery![4]

Today the medical community knows that there is no reason to rush in making vital decisions about breast cancer treatment. Today no woman should wake up with a surprise mastectomy. Instead she and her doctors have the time they need to decide on the proper treatment. Studies of her biopsy (pathology) can provide information about the makeup of the cancer cells involved and whether they are aggressive or slow-growing.

Today at least 50 percent of all women diagnosed with breast cancer can have their breast saved! Lumpectomy followed by radiation has proved as effective as mastectomy in treating cancer. But women, of course, must also know the negatives about this treatment before they decide which they want. Knowing is what this book is about.

Today we know that chemotherapy, given in adequate doses, can cut the rate of recurrence and raise the percentage of breast cancer survival. We know that drugs like tamoxifen can also reduce recurrence and prolong survival.

Also realize that you are already a little ahead of the game. You have been diagnosed. And from the day of that diagnosis you are considered a "breast cancer survivor."

It isn't always easy for a doctor to diagnose cancer from the many cysts and harmless lumps that are often present in our breasts. In fact, while false positives are extremely rare, failures to diagnose breast cancer are the second most frequent reason for patients suing doctors, according to a 1990 study by the Physicians Insurers Association.

Sometimes "the diagnosis was delayed because the physical findings failed to impress the physician, particularly when a mammogram was normal," according to William L. Donegan, M.D., of Sinai Samaritan Medical Center, writing in *The New England Journal of Medicine*.

A majority of these women were young and premenopausal. "The problem appears to lie in both a failure to appreciate the potential importance of a breast mass and the lack of a quick and convenient means for accurate diagnosis," Dr. Donegan wrote. This happens, he explained, because doctors know that most breast lumps will turn out to be benign and because biopsies take time and are expensive.

By touch, "Cysts cannot be distinguished reliably from solid masses," Dr. Donegan noted.[5]

But your diagnosis is "in." Now it's time to consider the options open to you.

First, some positive news: Breast cancer is *not* the number one killer of women. (That designation goes to heart disease.) Indeed, lung cancer, not breast cancer, is the number one cause of cancer death among women. More women develop breast cancer than lung cancer, but their survival chances are much greater. In 1990, for instance, 175,000 women were diagnosed with breast cancer while 44,500 died of the disease. In comparison, 60,000 women were diagnosed with lung cancer and 51,000 died in that year. By 1992 deaths from lung cancer had increased to 53,000. And if that's not enough to make you quit smoking, consider a new study that shows smokers with breast cancer have a greater chance of dying of the disease.[6]

There is more good news about breast cancer: The five-year survival rate for Stage I (very early) cancer is more than 90 percent, according to the National Cancer Institute. And in January 1995, Dr. Samuel Broder, the retiring director of the National Cancer Institute, announced that the latest data on cancer deaths from 1989-92 showed a "clear decline in deaths" from breast cancer for white women in almost every age group -- and an 18% decline for white women aged 30 to 39.[7]

But black women have not experienced this decline, and 46,000 women -- of all races, ages, and national origin -- are still likely to die of the disease within the next year. Nobody knows for sure which of us will make it and which won't. Who cares whether 90 percent of one group of women survived? You want to know about YOU!

REMEMBER, IT'S YOUR LIFE
You are ultimately responsible for what is done to you. And you must, like a good gambler, consider the odds and the options. Should you have a lumpectomy with radiation or a mastectomy? A mastectomy with immediate reconstruction? Are you a good candidate for tamoxifen? And when the biopsy has removed all of an encapsulated pre-cancer, there is sometimes even the option of having no additional treatment, just careful follow-up. In most cases, however, the less you do, the greater the chance of recurrence.

But perhaps your cancer is one of the slow-growing, non-aggressive kinds, or perhaps you have a tumor in situ (totally encapsulated) which some doctors regard as pre-cancerous. You have to find out what your options are. Knowledge is power. Knowledge is knowing the odds.

Even the best hospitals and doctors make mistakes. You have to be responsible for what is happening to you. Has someone forgotten your medicine? Do you feel unusual pain? Did the hospital give you a chest x-ray before any surgery requiring major anesthesia?

If your doctor has a mind-set about a particular treatment (breast conservation, mastectomy, etc.), get a second opinion. You should, if possible, get a second opinion on *everything*.

Whatever the stage of your treatment, make sure you are getting the best. Don't be afraid to complain if you feel your physician is not taking you seriously. Don't be afraid to ask questions. Don't be afraid to mention any problems that you are having or anything that the doctors or nurses may have overlooked at a given time.

You have the right to be afraid for your life and the quality of that life. Don't waste your fears on being scared of the people who are treating you!

KNOWLEDGE IS POWER

The purpose of this book is to give you some basic knowledge and the names of various resources that can help you cope and make the necessary decisions that otherwise will be made for you!

Know what you are up against. No doctor can say, "This will cure you." There are too many variables. You need to know the percentages and the options. Only if you prepare yourself, like the good gambler I mentioned earlier, will you make the best possible choice.

I can speak from experience on this matter. Years after my biopsy for a benign cyst, another suspicious area was discovered on a mammogram. This time the biopsy was "positive," a peculiar description for something I regarded as particularly negative. (And my cancer would NOT have been found without that mammogram.) This time I faced all the hard choices as well as the terror and fear of breast cancer. Now it seemed, I could lose a breast, my self-image, my hair, my feeling of well-being -- and my life. If the brave die but once and cowards many times, the anxious live our troubles times over. This book is written to help women like me accept the gamble, learn the odds, and act rationally, not with certainty that we will win, but with confidence that we have played our hands well.

While I was trying to sort out what to do, I was surprised at how difficult it was to get information on breast cancer. Even though I had excellent doctors, I couldn't find anything that put all the information I wanted in one place. And most books by breast cancer patients were written in the first person about very personal fears and experiences. I didn't want to know about their experiences as much as I wanted to get some facts about everything connected with the disease.

I have been surprised by the number of women I talked to who couldn't tell me what type of breast cancer they had. (There are some 15 different kinds.) Every woman facing breast cancer should know what she is dealing with. She should know what cards she is holding.

So, this book is not my story but what I learned along the way, and afterwards. I hope what I've written -- with the help of the experts I've consulted -- will assist you in dealing with the emotional and intellectual challenges that you face and in making the choices that will help you most. As a fellow gambler, I also wish you the best possible roll of the dice. (In the end, the treatment I chose was mastectomy with immediate reconstruction, followed by chemotherapy and then tamoxifen, which I'm still taking.)

There is far more information about breast cancer in this book than could have been put together just a few years ago. Even so, it is not intended to be a page-turner. You may find some of the information repeated in various chapters. That's intentional. If you've decided on a lumpectomy with radiation, you probably won't be interested in reading about mastectomy or reconstruction. If you have a ductal cancer in situ and don't need adjuvant chemotherapy, there's not much point in reading about how to cope with hair loss!

But do learn as much as you can. Let's play our hands with all the smarts we can acquire. Let's make decisions based on what will be best for us. Let's pray. Let's find lovers and friends and relatives to lean on, to share our experiences with, and to be helped by.

And let's get through the nights of terror and live again.

2. THE ODDS FOR BREAST CANCER SOME RISK FACTORS AND POSSIBLE PREVENTATIVES

The statistics for breast cancer risk seem to change almost as rapidly as the odds posted at the Kentucky Derby, and different studies can -- and often do -- come up with different results.

It's natural to want to find out why you or someone you love got breast cancer. It's easy even to put yourself at fault for doing something or not doing something that got you in this pickle. But this much is known about the disease: *At least* 70 percent (or it may be as high as 85 percent) of women who develop breast cancer don't have any of the risk factors, except perhaps age.

There is another side to this coin, however. As Dr. Sandra M. Swain, a Washington oncologist, put it to a group of breast cancer survivors during a discussion of the disease: "I think all women are at high risk."[8]

AGE FACTORS

Age is by far the greatest risk factor for developing breast cancer. About 80 percent of women with the disease are over 50, and the median age for diagnosis in the U.S. is 63. So, the younger you are, the less likely you are to have breast cancer. In 1989 only 6 percent of women diagnosed with breast cancer were under 40, and another 15 percent were in their forties. The chances are only one in 19,608 for a woman 25 or younger to develop the disease.

Breast cancer is, however, the leading cause of death among "young" women aged 40 to 44; one reason is that there are few other killer diseases of such younger women. Another is that cancer may grow more quickly in a younger person, as all cells do. Younger women often have more aggressive tumors and more lymph node involvement, but if the tumors are the same, young and old have a similar prognosis. Age alone should not determine therapy, according to a study at Case Western Reserve University in Cleveland, Ohio.[9]

The death rate from breast cancer in premenopausal women has fallen 10.2 percent in the last twenty years, and still more in the years since 1990, according to the National Cancer Institute. Unfortunately, the mortality rate for black women in the same age group has risen. Black women overall experience less breast cancer than white women, but the incidence rates are higher than average for young Afro-American women, the cancer is more apt to be aggressive, and the mortality rates are also worse. Older black women have a lower rate of breast cancer than the average, but their mortality rate has increased by 22 percent in the last 16 years.

In fact, black women have a 2.2 higher risk of dying from breast cancer. Researchers and community leaders are urging improved screening resources and educational techniques to turn around this tragic situation.

ONE IN EIGHT?

Shock reigned when the National Cancer Institute revised its odds of the chances of a woman developing breast cancer to "one in eight" over her lifetime.

Larry Kessler and Tom Reynolds of the National Cancer Institute wrote this explanation in a letter: "...if 800 female babies born today experience today's risk of getting breast cancer as they age, and also experience all other causes of death at the same rates that prevail today, we would expect 100 of these female babies to be diagnosed with breast cancer eventually. Some will live very long and others very short lives." In other words, the one in eight figure is a lifetime risk, not the risk for next year!

Age also plays a part in other aspects of a woman's life. Your chances of developing breast cancer are slightly higher if you began menstruation before age 12 or started menopause after age 55. The general consensus about this risk is that women who menstruate longer produce more estrogen, and this hormone, in turn, is one of the prime suspects in breast cancer development. More about this later.

The way estrogen is processed by a woman's body may provide a clue to her risk of developing breast cancer. The culprit is a component hormone or metabolite of natural estrogen that may promote abnormal cell growth. Women developing breast cancer seem to have a higher level of this metabolite. One day researchers may find a way to block production of this wayward hormone.

Teenage childbearing may present a lot of problems but produces at least one positive benefit: Women who have their first child before age 20 reduce their risk of breast cancer. On the other hand, women who have their first child at age 30 or older, or have no children, have an increased risk factor of almost 2 percent. (That doesn't mean, however, that a woman's chances of getting breast cancer increase to one in six nor does it mean she has two times the chance.)

Here's some good news: Breast feeding, the longer the better, seems to be a protective factor against breast cancer.

On the other hand, there is inconclusive evidence that induced abortion before age 45 increases breast cancer risk.

FAMILY HISTORY

Researchers have known for some time that a gene they call BRCA1 could be responsible for most familial breast cancer. Although scientists knew the gene resided somewhere in chromosome 17, the breakthrough came in the fall of 1994 when the National Institutes of Health held a special press conference to report that researchers in Utah and North Carolina were announcing in the upcoming issue of *Science* that they had isolated the gene. Women who inherit certain mutations of BRCA1 may have as much as an 85 percent chance of developing breast and/or ovarian cancer by age 70 and account for about percent of all breast cancer victims. Even with such inherited risk factors, however, each individual has a 50 percent chance that she *doesn't* carry this gene.

Scientists describe the work involved in identifying different mutations of this gene as "laborious," but it does bring researchers "one step closer to devising a test that will be useful in making prognostic tests," says Dr. Harold Varmus, head of the National Institutes of Health.[10] Eventually a simple blood test could be used by high risk women to see if they have a mutation of the gene.

Although there are some families where, tragically, breast cancer runs rampant because of inherited genetic factors, the risks for other women with a mother or sister with the disease are not nearly as great, more like a three-fold increase. Even this is not quite as scary as it sounds. As Dr. Susan Love noted in a television report on breast cancer, your lifetime risk might increase from 1 in 8 to 1 in 6. Nonetheless, a family history of breast cancer -- even involving cousins -- constitutes a risk factor. The possibility of recurrence also increases: Women with a first-degree (mother, sister) relative with breast cancer are more likely to have cancer recur in the other breast within three years of the original diagnosis.

A study of Utah families showed "...approximately 17% to 19% of breast cancer in the population could be attributed to family history," while the Nurses' Health Study has shown a family history in 6 percent.[11]

Familial risks may even cross the gender line. Women with first degree male relatives with prostate cancer also may have a greater risk of developing breast cancer, according to a study at the M.D. Anderson Cancer Center.[12]

BENIGN BREAST DISEASE

For many years benign breast disorders (usually lumped together in a category called "fibrocystic disease") were considered cancer risks in themselves. And even if you had a *benign* breast biopsy, the very fact that you had it was believed to increase your odds for breast cancer. But now the odds seem to be better on this front. Most "fibrocystic changes," the tenderness or lumps that come and go with the menstrual cycle, hormones and menopause, are generally no longer automatically assumed to be forerunners of breast cancers.

A Vanderbilt University study does suggest that one common benign breast growth, fibroadenoma, usually found in women in their twenties and thirties, may double the risk of later breast cancer, particularly if a woman has a family history of the disease. If you do have a breast biopsy and the tissue is benign, your risk factors for cancer may not be changed much, according to some new findings. Some abnormal tissue conditions may indicate a slight risk increase, but they aren't even precancerous. The only condition associated with a definite higher risk factor is atypical hyperplasia, which means there are too many cells (hyperplasia) and that they are unusual (atypical). Atypical hyperplasia should be carefully watched, especially if the patient has a family history of breast cancer or other abnormalities such as microcalcifications on mammograms, according to Dr. Mark A. Helvie, speaking at a University of Michigan Medical School symposium.[13]

ESTROGEN AND OTHER HORMONES

There is no question that the hormone estrogen plays a part in breast cancer. Many of these cancers, for instance, are "estrogen receptive"; that is, they need estrogen to grow.

Estrogen is even under suspicion for the increased incidence of breast cancer over the last few decades because women now manufacture the hormone for a much longer period of time. Two hundred years ago, the average age for the onset of menstruation was 17, and some women went into menopause as early as age 35. Today the averages are more like 13 and 52. And, since women have fewer children today, they don't have the "rest" periods that pregnancy gives.

Before estrogen replacement therapy (ERT) became common, women who had their ovaries removed before age 35 were considered to have one third the breast cancer risk of women with later, natural menopause.

Birth control pills, which contain both estrogen and progesterone hormones, seem to protect against ovarian cancer, and new studies find little increase of breast cancer among women taking "the pill" for ten years or longer.[14] The consensus seems to be that, unless there is long-term use, any risk drops rapidly once the drugs are stopped, while the increased protection against ovarian cancer continues for some ten years. But not everyone agrees with this theory.

A recent report from the Nurses' Health Study indicates that estrogen replacement therapy, particularly when given with progesterone, does increase breast cancer risk, especially for those over 55 using the therapy for five or more years.[15] On the other hand, an analysis of 13 studies since 1979 has shown a 35 percent reduction in coronary heart disease and death among users of [unopposed] estrogen.[16] Heart disease kills more women annually than all cancers.

Estrogen not only reduces hot flashes, but helps protect women against heart disease, reduces vaginal dryness, and provides some protection against osteoporosis. And now scientists undertaking studies to see if some breast cancer survivors, especially younger premenopausal women, would actually benefit from ERT!

LIFESTYLE: WEIGHT, DIET, ALCOHOL

Although there have been numerous studies attempting to link such no-no's as fat intake, obesity, cigarettes, and alcohol to breast cancer, the results have ranged from negative to inconclusive.

• Cigarettes cause lung cancer, but they don't cause breast cancer. Hair dyes and tranquilizers are also off the hook.

• Although postmenopausal fat women have a slightly higher risk of breast cancer (and their prognosis may be worsened by fat-associated diseases), there seems to be a reduced incidence of breast cancer in premenopausal fatties! Being fatter before forty may pose greater risk later: A recent study showed that weight gain in a woman's twenties to around thirty, even as little as 10 or 20 pounds, may increase the risk of later breast cancer.[17]

• Researchers are looking into the effects of teenagers' diet and fat intake on long-range cancer risk. But, although breast cancer rates are lower in some countries with less fat consumption, such as Japan, researchers have been unable to come up with solid proof that fat is at fault.

• Some studies do link an increased risk of breast cancer to even a limited intake of alcohol, but others don't. At a recent American Cancer Society National Conference, however, two doctors agreed that although alcohol is not a major risk for breast cancer, it is one that can be eliminated by abstinence.[18]

And one NCI research project found alcohol raised the levels of several hormones in premenopausal women, which may link alcohol with breast cancer. Meanwhile, research in this area continues.

But before you abandon drinking forever, listen to what one scientist, Dr. Eugene Pergament, told the *Chicago Tribune* about alcohol and breast cancer risk. "In France it took 17 drinks per week to bring about a tripling of basic risk," he said, calling alcohol "another shibboleth" [catchword] in terms of risk factors.[19]

ENVIRONMENTAL FACTORS

In a Mt. Sinai School of Medicine study, that nasty pesticide of the past, DDT, was linked to breast cancer. But a large study by researchers at the Kaiser Foundation Research Institute in Oakland, California, found no DDT-breast cancer link.[20]

Studies by the National Institutes of Health and others are also being undertaken to determine what other environmental elements could be risk factors for breast cancers, including industrial chemicals called polychlorinated biphenyls (PCB's), exhaust fumes, contaminants in food and water, electro-magnetic fields, chemicals formed from high temperature cooking, endogenous retroviruses and artificial (nighttime) light! Scientists are also trying to answer this question: Is it possible that some of these environmental chemicals function in some way as hormones?

MAMMOGRAPHY

Is mammography itself a risk? The procedure does involve a low level of radiation, and one Canadian study startled doctors (and patients) by indicating a higher risk of death in women aged 40 to 49 who had received mammograms. Some scientists have pointed out that the Canadian study involved mammograms made with "older" machinery and only one view of the breast. And other studies show no such risk.

The recent controversies surrounding this age group and mammograms also involve the possibility that mammograms do not work as well for younger women, whose breast tissue is much denser, making problems more difficult to spot. According to the National Cancer Institute,[21] at least two studies indicate that these younger women have substantially benefitted from mammograms. Even so, the NCI recommendations for mammograms for women under 50 now include only those at high risk. On the other hand, the American Cancer Society advises that women aged 40 to 49 have a mammogram at least every two years, and my bet is that eventually this recommendation will be adopted by the medical community.

Mammograms for women over 50 on the other hand, have definitely improved mortality rates in that age group. Some scientists suggest that having mammograms should relate to a woman's menopausal status rather than to her age and begin when she starts to experience "change of life," rather than when she reaches 50.

GEOGRAPHY

What part does geography play in the development of breast cancer? Why, for example, is there a higher risk in some Northeast and Middle Atlantic states in the US? Why is breast cancer so much more common in many industrialized nations? We don't know...yet.

There are intensive studies underway to learn about the biology of cancer in general and the genetics of breast tumors in particular. Exciting discoveries have been made, including the identification of a breast cancer gene, BRCA1 (for Breast Cancer 1). As mentioned earlier in this chapter, women who inherit the mutation of this gene appear to be at much greater risk. The next steps are to develop ways both of testing for mutations of this gene and finding strategies to prevent the cancer from developing in susceptible women.

Dr. James D'Angelo, an oncologist and hematologist practicing in the Washington, D.C., area, believes that the cure for cancer will come through genetic engineering. "Cancer is a cell that no longer responds to the normal body processes that control growth. The solution is through genetic engineering -- to make it a cell that will respond," he says.

BRCA1 is not the only genetic suspect in breast cancer by a long shot. Other prognostic markers include mutations of the genes P53 and c-myc, and the HER2/neu (c-*erb*B-2) oncogene protein, which, if damaged, can cause more aggressive cancer. Researchers are investigating genetic markers and genetic suppression, along with the role of viruses, and the possibility of developing vaccines against various forms of the disease.

Denser than normal breast tissue is another possible risk factor. "It could be that breast density is a marker of past exposure that contributes to breast cancer's development or produces a susceptible condition," according to Dr. Celia Byrne in the *Journal of the National Cancer Institute*.[22] Hormones might be able to lower the density in high-risk women.

Angiogenesis (formation of new blood vessels), associated with a poorer prognosis in women who have these vessels in cancerous tumors, may also pose a risk for women with fibrocystic breast disease.[23]

There are so many unanswered questions. Why do certain families have a predisposition to breast cancer? Why are women with high socio-economic status at higher risk, regardless of race? Why do native Hawaiians and American Indians have the lowest risk of breast cancer in the United States? There is even some evidence that height may play a part in breast cancer. You name it, somebody is conducting a study. Then there is. . .

. . .STRESS

Ask a doctor about what role stress plays in the development of cancer, and there is a good chance he or she will say, "There is no real evidence that stress plays any role." Then, after a pause, some doctors will continue: "However, in my own experience..." And you'll hear a tale about a relative or friend or patient of the doctor's who developed cancer after a period of sustained or extreme stress.

And why not? Studies have already shown that the surviving spouse is at much greater risk for death for a year after the loss of the marriage partner (regardless of the cause of the partner's death). The immune system doesn't seem to work as well after such a loss. So, why wouldn't the same be true for other forms of stress?

Stress as a cause of illness is under study at the National Institute of Mental Health, now a part of the National Institutes of Health.

Dr. Susan J. Blumenthal, then chief of preventative and behavioral research at NIMH told *The Washington Post*: "Clinicians have long observed there are important mind-body interactions, and the public believes it strongly. But we've been missing the scientific underpinnings to explain them and scientists have been unable or unwilling to explore them."[24]

OUNCES OF PREVENTION

Some doctors have prescribed a drug, tamoxifen, used in breast cancer treatment, to help prevent the cancer in women at high risk for the disease. Tamoxifen blocks the formation of the estrogen involved in breast cancer disease but acts as an estrogen in other parts of the body. Tamoxifen, for example, seems to protect women against the loss of bone mass, just as estrogen replacement therapy protects postmenopausal women.

In 1992 a clinical trial was set up to study the use of the drug in healthy women with high breast cancer risk. In 1994 the trial ran into stormy waters. Among other things, it is part of the ongoing National Surgical Adjuvant Breast & Bowel Project which came under fire when faulty data was found in some of its studies. Anxiety levels about tamoxifen were raised when one of the previous trials, involving the use of tamoxifen or a placebo in women diagnosed with breast cancer, showed a higher incidence of endometrial (uterine) cancer in the tamoxifen group, as well as four deaths, an unusually high percentage for uterine cancer. This study also found the risk of uterine cancer to be much greater in women over 50 taking the drug.[25]

Although the same study showed that tamoxifen did reduce the recurrence of breast cancer by as much as 46%, the number of deaths was unusually high for endometrial (uterine) cancer, and there was some concern that tamoxifen might sometimes cause a more virulent form of the disease. The British journal, *The Lancet*, also published results of studies showing that tamoxifen use increased the risk of endometrial cancer, that the risk increased with length of use, and that tamoxifen takers showed more uterine abnormalities.[26]

Was it fair, critics asked, to have healthy women take a drug which might possibly give them another form of cancer?

The American tamoxifen "chemoprevention" trial with healthy women was started in 1992 at 270 centers in 47 states with a goal of including 16,000 participants. About half that number were enrolled in the study when the National Cancer Institute suspended enrollment. Later the NCI decided to continue enrollments because the possible benefits far exceeded the risk. By the summer of 1994 a Food and Drug Administration advisory panel voted to let the chemoprevention tamoxifen trial continue without major changes.

Half the women participating will receive daily doses of the real thing; i.e., 20 milligrams of tamoxifen, and half will take "fake" pills, or placebos, for five years. Only women with increased risk for breast cancer (those with a history of first-degree relatives with the disease, early menstruation, breast biopsies, no children or first child after age 30) or who are aged 60 or older have been considered for this large study. Scientists also hope to find out more about the effects of tamoxifen on heart disease and bone density.

DIET

In spite of the lack of evidence that fat is a risk factor, the gut reaction of many prominent oncologists is that fat is bad.

Some even recommend very low fat diets to patients. For one thing, fat cells produce estrogen, a known breast-cancer risk factor.

The "good fat" of the hour is olive oil. Already known to help raise high density lipoids (HDL), the "good" cholesterol, use of this oil may also help to reduce breast cancer development, according to at least one study.

It's a good idea for women to follow the National Cancer Institute's dietary guidelines, which recommend a low fat diet with at least five fruits and vegetables a day as well as plenty of fiber.

According to an editorial in the Institute's *Journal*,[27] 80 percent of 175 studies involving the relationship between fruits and vegetables (or their antioxidant equivalents) and cancer "have showed statistical significance. For no other risk factor besides smoking are the data as consistent and abundant."

Scientists at the Johns Hopkins University in Baltimore have found that sulforaphane, a compound in broccoli, blocked the growth of breast tumors in rats and helped control any tumors that did develop. Broccoli is a cruciferous vegetable, like its cousins cauliflower, Brussels sprouts, and cabbage. And there are very few calories in any of them.[28] Bon appetit!

There may be definitive answers down the road about the effects of diet and hormones. The National Institutes of Health has launched the Women's Health Initiative, the largest clinical trial ever undertaken in the United States. Part of the study will involve 160,000 postmenopausal women aged 50 to 79 from all ethnic and racial groups. They will be followed for 15 years in controlled studies to see what effects such factors as estrogen replacement therapy, low-fat diets, and calcium and vitamin D supplements have on the development of breast and colon cancer and heart disease.

And speaking of diet, mothers-to-be and those with newborn babies should know that a study published in

Epidemiology showed women who were breast-fed as babies were 26% less likely to develop breast cancer.[29]

VITAMINS, MINERALS, AND TRACE ELEMENTS

Fruits and vegetables are major sources of antioxidants, substances that prevent or control the effects of oxygen in cells and elsewhere. Antioxidants such as Vitamins C and E and beta carotene have been credited with cancer-fighting properties, as have folic acid, fiber, and other nutrients. One NCI study showed a decreased risk of colon cancer in women eating fruit fiber.

A study recently completed in China was the first to show hard evidence that vitamins and other supplements could reduce cancer. Of the 300,000 participants, those who had a daily dose of Vitamin E, beta carotene, and selenium had a 13 percent lower risk of death from cancer than those taking a placebo or other combinations of vitamins and minerals. (The Chinese in this study had vitamin-poor diets to begin with, however, as well as stomach cancer rates among the highest in the world.)[30]

Beta carotene lost some of the shine on its halo, and supplements suffered a setback, when a study of Finnish smokers showed a higher (18%) development of lung cancer in smokers taking beta carotene than in those who didn't. Smokers taking Vitamin E had a slightly higher rate of hemorrhagic stroke.[31]

Then another study, this one of patients with colon polyps (often precursors of colon cancer) found no difference in cancer development between groups taking either (1) beta carotene, (2) Vitamins C and E, (3) all three supplements and (4) only placebos.

But there always seems to be another side to the story. A recent study showed not only an increased risk of dying of breast cancer among patients with a high fat intake before diagnosis, but a slightly reduced risk of dying of the disease when patients increased their intake of beta carotene and vitamin C after diagnosis.[32]

Another ongoing study of 22,000 doctors, half of whom are taking beta carotene and half of whom aren't, will end in late 1995. Although this 12-year study has already shown the benefits of taking aspirin to prevent heart attacks and colon cancer, no such positive results have so far been released on the beta carotene front. (See Clinical Trials chapter.)

Supplements (or "micronutrients" as they are sometimes called) may possibly counteract the effects of meat-rich diets and even alcohol. But it's more important to eat plenty of fruits, vegetables and fibers, since scientists don't know which "micronutrients" might actually help prevent cancer. Some people feel comfortable taking extra Vitamin C and E, beta carotene, baby aspirin, and even selenium and other trace elements. If you do take such substances, make sure you don't overdo; some of them can be toxic in large doses. It's better to get your vitamins and minerals from *food*.

CLEAN LIVING

There is a possibility that exercise, combined with a high fiber diet, may reduce some estrogen levels, while alcohol and overweight increase the estrogen amounts in the blood. In other words, perhaps exercise can help and alcohol may hinder.

Exercise may be particularly important in reducing breast cancer in premenopausal women under age 40, according to a study reported in the *Journal of the National Cancer Institute*. "Our results suggest that implementation of regular exercise programs as a critical component of a healthy lifestyle should be a high priority for adolescent and adult women," researchers concluded.[33] Although women who exercised fairly strenuously four or more hours a week benefited the most, even those who had as little as two or three hours of exercise a week showed lower rates of breast cancer.

Mammograms

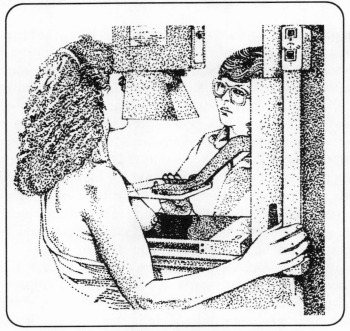

Technician positions patient for mammogram.
Figure courtesy FDA Consumer magazine.

Mammograms have proven their effectiveness in women 50 years of age and older, with research indicating a potential reduction of 30 to 40 percent in the death rate from breast cancer in that age group.

But the idea of annual or bi-annual mammograms for women 40 to 49 proved more controversial and has been modified by the National Cancer Institute, although this argument is far from over. Almost everyone agrees, however, that at the minimum all women over 40 should receive an annual clinical exam, that those aged 50 to 75 should have a yearly mammogram in addition to such an exam, and that women under 50 in high risk categories (personal history of breast cancer, a mother, sister or daughter with breast cancer, no children by age 30) should continue to have regular mammograms. Many in the medical community feel that older women should continue to have mammograms throughout their lifetime, no matter what their age. Meanwhile, the American Cancer Society has stood firm in its recommendation that women in their forties have a mammogram every one to two years.

Make sure that the place where you have your mammogram is accredited by the American College of Radiology and the facilities approved by the U.S. Food and Drug Administration. Doing this will assure you of both quality x-rays and readings. Mammography poses little threat in terms of radiation, but women previously treated with radiation for benign breast conditions (before we knew better) may have a greater risk of later developing breast cancer.

Researchers at universities in the USA and the Netherlands have demonstrated that breast cancer often grows twice as fast in women in their 40s, compared to older women. *New York Times* columnist Jane E. Brody noted that, "...as medical researchers have come to better understand the biology of breast cancer in younger women, many have concluded that for mammography to achieve its maximum life saving benefits, women under 50 should have the x-ray examination more often, rather than less often, than those over 50."[34]

Malcolm Gladwell echoed these sentiments in a scathing article in *The New Republic*: "In women in their 40s, however, tumors appear to grow much faster, and a mammogram typically provides only an eighteen-to-thirty-month early warning. In this group, anything other than an annual mammogram will give cancers a chance to grow and spread before they can be picked up."[35]

SUMMARY

To sum up: Live in moderation, have children early in life (if possible) and breast-feed them, exercise, avoid environmental toxins if you can, have regular breast exams, and, of course (!) do regular breast exams yourself every month. And remember to eat your vegetables.

3. DIAGNOSTIC TECHNIQUES

Perhaps you have just had a mammogram and there are suspicious flecks (microcalcifications) on it, or perhaps you have a lump that your doctor feels needs investigation. What will happen? If your doctor feels strongly that the suspicious area may turn out to be cancer, he or she may tell you to stop birth control or menopausal hormone replacement therapy until the diagnostic tests are completed. (These hormones may affect cancer development and growth.)

The next step, of course, is to find out if there really *is* cancer present and if so, how far it has developed, and what kind it is. Part of the good news about breast cancer today is that it can often be more easily detected. Thanks to mammograms, more cancers found today while they are still small. Through analysis of suspicious tissue removed (biopsy), physicians called pathologists can find out how aggressive the cancer is and whether it is hormone-receptive; i.e., is the cancer stimulated by the hormones estrogen or progesterone or both. Positive readings can make a difference in deciding whether to use hormone treatments.

And blood tests can sometimes detect whether the cancer has spread.

The medical profession's diagnostic tools for finding and evaluating breast cancer include the following:

1. MAMMOGRAMS

Mammograms are sophisticated x-rays of the breast. They can show cysts, masses, tumors too small to be felt, and calcifications, or a gathering of calcium salts in a part of the breast tissue. Ironically, large calcifications are usually considered harmless, but tiny microscopic deposits, called microcalcifications, sometimes cluster around cancer cells. Many "in situ" lesions and cancers much too small to be felt (or palpitated) are now picked up by mammography. Such cancers have a very high cure rate.

These low-power, sophisticated x-rays are particularly useful in finding cancer in older women, whose breasts are fatter. (Younger or childless women are apt to have more fibrous tissue in their breasts, making them denser and harder to evaluate.) Mammograms are also used as a guide in a diagnostic procedure called "needle localization biopsy," where the suspicious area cannot be felt or is deep inside the breast. (See Types of Biopsy.)

2. ULTRASOUND

Ultrasound, or sonograms, are high-frequency sound waves. These high frequency waves are sent into the breast and the pattern of echoes from the waves shows up on a monitor, similar to a TV screen. Ultrasound can also be used as a guide in needle biopsies.

3. BIOPSY

A biopsy is the removal of suspicious tissue, fluids or cells, which are then examined and evaluated by a pathologist.

Depending on what type it is, you may have your biopsy in a doctor's office, or in a clinic or hospital. A simple needle biopsy ("needle aspiration"), where the physician or surgeon draws fluid from the suspicious area, can be done in the office without any anesthetic. An "excisional," or complete biopsy, on the other on hand, may require hospitalization and anesthesia. Even with this type of biopsy, however, you are usually treated on an "outpatient" basis, and are in and out of the hospital on the same day.

Some biopsies produce pain for a day or so after surgery. If you have a biopsy and experience pain, ask for pain medicine.   Some physicians are reluctant to prescribe pain medicine, partly because they were schooled in the terrors of drug addiction.   You are highly unlikely to get addicted to anything by taking a couple of pain pills.   Insist on them if you are in pain.

TYPES OF BIOPSY

Incisional Biopsy

In this kind of biopsy, only part of the suspicious area is removed for examination.

Excisional Biopsy

The entire lump or suspicious area is removed as well as a small area around it.   The outer edges of the biopsied area are called the "margins."

Frozen Section

This is a quick test for cancer cells done by freezing portions of the tissue that has been removed.   (In the "old" days -- about 10 or 15 years ago! -- the surgeon would wait for a report on the frozen section, and, if cancer were found, immediately perform a mastectomy while the patient was still under anesthesia.)   Although surgeons still ask for frozen section biopsies, the test results are less accurate than those from a "permanent" section, and further treatment now usually is delayed until the results of *all* tests are in, and the patient and doctor have had a chance to study and discuss all the options available.

Permanent Section

This is a more accurate and detailed method of examining the tissue for cancer.   The procedure is much more time-consuming than a frozen section, but the pathologist discovers much   more   about   the   tissue,   including   what   its   cell characteristics are, what kinds of cancer cells, if any, are present, whether they have aggressive qualities, and what the hormone factors are.

TYPES OF BIOPSY PROCEDURES

Needle Aspiration
The physician uses a needle to suction out fluid or tissue from the lump or suspicious area. Sometimes ultrasound is used to guide the needle to the site of the aspiration. Afterwards a pathologist examines the material removed.

Wide-bore Needle Biopsy
If the lump being examined is solid, the physician may use a needle with a sharp point to cut out a portion of the tissue for the pathologist to examine.

Needle Localization Biopsy
Technicians use mammograms to pinpoint the exact location of the suspicious area. Employing the mammograms as a guide, the technician then inserts a needle into the breast. Another mammogram is taken to make sure the needle is in the right place. If it is, a wire is inserted in the breast which the surgeon uses as a guideline for performing the biopsy. This procedure is often done under anesthesia in a hospital, but the patient usually goes home the same day.

This type of biopsy is no fun: You must remain very still during the mammography parts of the process and it may hurt. If your surgeon schedules you for such a biopsy, with anesthesia, try to get it done early in the day. The reason for an early start is that you will be unable to eat or drink anything because you are going to have anesthesia, so you'll be more comfortable having the whole thing over with as soon as possible.

Sterotactic Automated Large-core Biopsy

The patient lies face down on a special table with her breast protruding through a large hole. From this position, mammograms are taken to determine the exact location of the lump or suspicious area. Then a computer-guided needle goes to the spot and extracts a tissue sample. This biopsy, less painful and requiring less tissue, is "great technology" and may herald "tremendous changes in the next few years," according to surgeon James Wolcott. He cautions, however, that this procedure cannot be used for every biopsy. "I'm selective," he says. And the technology itself doesn't yet work for lesions close to the muscle, the nipple, or under the arm.

WHAT THE BIOPSY CAN TELL

The pathologist can tell much more from a biopsy than whether the tissue has cancer cells, and the list is growing every day. He or she can also determine what kinds of cancer the cells contain and whether they have aggressive components. Such information is becoming more and more important in deciding on treatment options.

Hormone Receptors

With enough tissue sample, the pathologist can determine if the cancer cells are estrogen and/or progesterone receptive (or positive). "Estrogen positive" is good because it means that the cells need estrogen to grow, and so physicians can use anti-estrogen drugs such as tamoxifen as a weapon to inhibit cell growth. If the tumor is "estrogen negative," anti-estrogen drugs aren't likely to work, although tamoxifen may help most postmenopausal women regardless. Postmenopausal women are also more likely to be estrogen-positive.

"Progesterone positive" means that the cells need progesterone to grow. The best prognosis is to be both estrogen and progesterone positive; drugs like tamoxifen seem to work better in this situation.

DNA and Other Measurements

DNA analysis of the tissue can measure the "flow cytometry," or the total DNA content in a tumor sample. If the cells have the right amount of DNA, they are "diploid"; if the DNA is abnormal, the cells are "aneuploid" and are generally more aggressive. The S-Phase measures the growth rate of the tumor, the number of cells manufacturing new DNA at any time before they divide. If the S-Phase is low, the tumor may be less aggressive.

Other measures include oncogenes such as c-*erb*B-2 (also called HER-2/neu). If a tumor contains a high level of the c-*erb*B-2 oncogene, the prognosis for recurrence may be worse. In a recent study, women with positive lymph nodes and high levels of c-*erb*B-2 responded best when treated with high doses of chemotherapy that included Adriamycin. An example might be CAF (the cyclophosphamide, Adriamycin and fluorouracil combination), while women without this genetic factor seemed to respond better to the less potent CMF (cyclophosphamide, methotrexate and fluorouracil) combination.[36] (See Adjuvant Chemotherapy chapter for more information on this.)

The tumor cells will also be examined under a microscope to see how normal (differentiated) or abnormal (undif-ferentiated) they appear.

Through an inking process, the pathologist also determines if the cancer cells go to the edge or "margin" of the tumor removed. If the margins are clear, there is a better chance that no cancer remains in the breast.

The protein p53 appears to play a two-faced role in prognosis. On the one hand, a normal form of p53 may suppress tumor development, while an abnormal, or mutated form, may indicate a worse prognosis.

THE LYMPH NODES

Breast cancer is most likely to spread first to the lymph nodes under the arm. This spread is called "axillary-node metastasis," so, except for in situ cases, surgeons routinely remove some or all of the nodes as a diagnostic procedure to see if there has been any cancer spread. If the nodes are involved but the cancer hasn't spread anywhere else, the condition is called "regional metastasis."

The number of lymph nodes with any cancer cells helps determine the extent of the cancer and how it will be treated ("Staging"). If all the nodes are clear and other prognostic factors are good, the patient may not have to have any additional treatment.

The removal of all, or even some, of the lymph nodes, is called "axillary node dissection." This procedure, done under anesthesia, is a relatively major surgical event, requiring insertion of a drain under your arm for several days. Most surgeons don't mention that patients will experience post-surgical numbness and swelling and must exercise the affected arm to restore normal use. (See Lymph Node Surgery.)

NUCLEAR MEDICINE, X-RAYS, ETC.

If you are diagnosed as having breast cancer, you will almost certainly have a chest x-ray, just to make sure the cancer has not spread to the chest area. The doctor may also order other tests, including bone and liver scans, the other places to which most breast cancer spreads. A metastatic workup may include other tests as well. Most of these tests involve "nuclear medicine," that is, a radioactive material is inserted in the veins so that the scanner can pick up images. A "CAT" scan (computerized axial tomography, also called CT), uses pencil-like x-ray beams to look inside the body. An MRI ("Magnetic resonance imaging") machine uses electromagnets to look inside the body. The major complaint about these tests (besides their expense) is that patients often feel claustrophobic when they are required to remain very still in a small covered space while the procedure is administered. Some of the tests are noisy as well.

Ultrasound, another diagnostic tool already discussed, employs high-frequency sound waves to produce images on a TV-like screen.

BLOOD AND OTHER TESTS

Your blood tells a lot about you, and scientists are able to "read" blood samples to find out, for example, if your red and white blood cells are normal and if your kidney and liver functions are okay. A "tumor test" for the presence of carcinoembroyonic antigen (CEA) is effective over 50% of the time in helping to determine if there has been any cancer metastasis.[37]

Other possible prognostic indicators include Cathepsin (a cell surface measurement) and the identification of tiny metastases in the bone marrow. New, tiny blood vessels (tumor angiogenesis) near the site of the cancer may mean a more aggressive growth. According to the *Journal of the National Cancer Institute,*[38] there is some indication that patients with ductal cancer in situ (see following chapter) may have a greater risk of cancer progression if such microblood vessels are involved.

But now, in your case, the analysis is over. Based on what is known about your cancer, it's time for you and your doctors to consider the treatment options.

4. WHAT BREAST CANCER IS: TYPES AND STAGING

Most of us know some breast basics -- aside from being a sex object, the breast produces milk. And, from time to time, all of us have experienced breast fullness or pain during the menstrual cycle.

Now, however, it's time to learn some basic facts about what the breast is composed of and where, in most cases, breast cancer develops.

Although the breast is largely fatty tissue, it is also complex, because of its primary function -- supplying milk. So it has thousands of cells whose job is to secrete that substance, on demand. Every month, during a woman's menstrual cycle, the breast goes through several hormonal changes. If there is no pregnancy, the menstrual cycle starts again. If there is a pregnancy, the breast prepares itself for the milking job ahead.

To accomplish this miraculous feat, the breast has 15 to 20 "lobes," or glands, which secrete the milk. Each lobe has smaller sections called "lobules." The lobes and lobules are connected by small tubes, or "ducts," which carry milk to the nipple. (The area around the nipple is the "areola" and contains sweat glands and hair follicles.)

Ninety percent of all breast cancers start in the ducts or lobes of the breast.

Picture, if you will, a small circle. Inside the circle are smaller circles, the cancer cells, which spend their time multiplying within their home circle (the tumor). Imagine this circle inside a duct. As long as the inmates of that circle, the cancer cells, remain inside their circle home, they are, medically speaking, "in situ," the Latin for "in place." Some researchers believe that many women who die at a ripe old age from some unrelated condition will have some ductal in situ cancer that has never spread or even been detected.

But many of us won't be that lucky.

Unfortunately, sometimes things get very crowded inside the cells' circle home, and they break out. Once they're out, they travel in search of new homes -- in other ducts. If the cells spread from a duct, the condition is called "invasive ductal carcinoma," or "infiltrating intraductal carcinoma." If the cells start and spread from the lobes, the condition is known as infiltrating lobular carcinoma. If left untreated, the cells can spread to the lymph nodes under the arm or those under the breast bone, or through the blood stream, and from there to other parts of the body.

The following is a brief description of the major types of breast cancer. Sometimes more than one type of cancer may be present.

DUCTAL

Often referred to as intraductal carcinoma, this cancer starts in the ducts of the breast and accounts for about 75 percent of the all breast cancers. Ductal cancer is usually only found in one breast. If ductal cancer is found early, before it spreads, or becomes "invasive" in the breast, the prognosis is very good. (More about this under Stages.)

If ductal cancer spreads, it usually goes first to the lymph nodes under the arm, and sometimes to the nodes beneath the breast bone. It can reappear on the skin in the breast area or nearby tissue and sometimes spreads to the breast bone itself. This kind of spread is called "regional" because it is in the same area as the original disease was. (If the cancer reappears on the chest after a mastectomy to the area, the condition is considered more serious.) If cancer spreads beyond the local

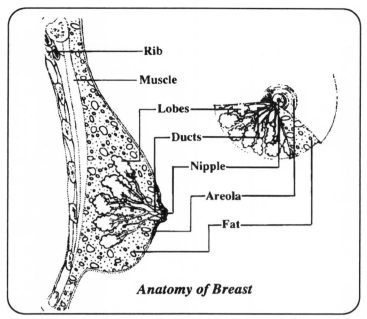

Anatomy of Breast

area, it generally goes to the bones, brain, liver, lungs, or the central nervous system.

LOBULAR

Also known as lobular carcinoma, this cancer starts in the breast lobes and is more often found in both breasts than other types of cancer. There is also a greater chance that it will recur in the other breast. Much lobular cancer is "in situ"; that is, it hasn't spread anywhere and sometimes doesn't even have any tumor, or mass, that can be identified. The problem with this very early cancer is that it is apt to recur and become "invasive" at a later time.

About 25 to 35 percent of women with LCIS will develop an invasive cancer in the same area, often many years later.

Unlike ductal cancer, if the lobular type spreads through the body, it will generally attack the membranes, or the thin coverings of such areas as the lining of the brain or the pericardial sac that surrounds the heart.

INFLAMMATORY

This is an uncommon but fast-moving cancer in which the breast is warm, red, and swollen, and the skin may resemble an orange peel. The breast's color and warmth is caused by cancer cells blocking the lymph vessels in the breast. Because this cancer can spread rapidly, it is usually treated aggressively. Luckily, it only accounts for 1 to 2 percent of all breast cancer, and the five-year survival rate, once only 2 percent, is now about 40 percent.[39]

PAGET'S DISEASE AND EPITHELIOMA

These are cancers of the nipple. In Paget's disease there is the oozing and crusting similar to what you'd find with dermatitis. Paget's disease probably starts in a duct. Because of its location, treatment has usually been removal of the breast (mastectomy). Now this disease is often treated by removing only the nipple and the areola (the colored area around the nipple), and following up with radiation therapy.

TUBULAR BREAST CANCER

This cancer gets its name because the cancer cells look like -- you guessed it -- little tubes. The outlook for tubular breast cancer is good because it is "well differentiated" and generally does not spread to the lymph nodes under the arm. This type of tumor accounts for about 2 percent of all breast cancer.

MEDULLARY BREAST CANCER

"A big gray glob" is the way Joyce Wadler described her mostly medullary tumor in her book *My Breast*.[40] Named for its resemblance to brain tissue (medulla), medullary accounts for about 5 to 7 percent of breast cancers and has a good outlook for cure; that is, the five year survival rate is higher than that for infiltrating ductal carcinoma. One recent study showed black women twice as likely to develop medullary carcinoma. Sometimes the medullary cancer may also show ductal carcinoma characteristics; then the prognosis is less good.

MUCINOUS
This is a slow-growing cancer which manufactures mucus. Although it can become quite large, this cancer has a good prognosis and accounts for around 3 percent of all breast cancers.

OTHER
Other, rarer forms of breast cancer include papillary, secretory, apocrine and metaplastic. In all, there are about 15 types of breast cancer.

BREAST CANCER STAGING AND POSSIBLE TREATMENTS

Most types of cancer are divided into "stages," or levels of severity based on tumor size and the extent of any growth outside of the original location. Each stage has its own treatment options as well as a lettering system (**TNM**) to describe the cancer: **T** stands for the tumor and its size, **N** for whether the cancer has spread to the local lymph nodes and **M** for whether it has spread, or metastasized, to other parts of the body.

Breast cancer is divided into several stages: "In Situ," Stage I, Stages IIA & IIB, Stages IIIA & IIIB, and Stage IV. If you had the very earliest or "in situ" breast cancer, the abbreviation would be **TIS** (for Tumor In Situ), **NO** (zero lymph nodes involved) and **MO** (zero distant metastasis).

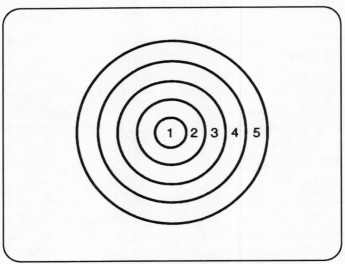

Tumor sizes are measured in centimeters.
A one-inch tumor would be about 2.5 centimeters.
Figure courtesy FDA Consumer magazine.

A person with Stage II breast cancer and an inch-sized tumor (2.5 centimeters) with an underarm lymph node showing some cancer cells would have these initials: T2 (the tumor is between 2 and 5 centimeters), N1 (positive lymph node), and M0 (no metastasis).

Although staging is still important, today the medical community recognizes there are other factors to be considered. If, for example, a patient diagnosed as Stage I (very early with a small tumor and no lymph node involvement) has a cancer showing many aggressive features, she will be treated differently from a patient with no negative prognostic features.

Similarly, a patient with Stage IIB disease whose tumor is barely over 2 centimeters, with one lymph node involved and good pathological prognostic features, will be treated far differently from a patient with 10 positive lymph nodes and an aggressive form of the disease!

But doctors have to start somewhere, and staging is one way to begin.

INTRADUCTAL OR DUCTAL CANCER IN SITU
Tis, NO, MO

Some physicians believe that ductal cancer in situ should be treated as a pre-malignancy, because all the cells are encapsulated -- that is, they haven't spread out of the original small area. (As mentioned earlier, "in situ" means "in place" in Latin.)

The treatment of choice for this condition is often lumpectomy (removal of the cancer and some of the tissue around it), followed by radiation therapy. The advantage of a lumpectomy is, of course, that it preserves the breast. Follow-up radiation is important: In a clinical trial, five-year "event free" survival rates for women with intraductal cancer in situ were better when they received radiation therapy.[41] This improvement (84.4 percent versus 73.8 percent) was due almost entirely to a reduction in the recurrence of cancer in the same breast.

Because mammography sometimes finds these cancers when they are very small, they may also be treated by a biopsy alone, followed by radiation. The biopsy would have to be one which removed sufficient tissue or "margins" around the tumor to catch any malingering cancer cells.

Another possible treatment is partial or total mastectomy (removal of the breast). This procedure might be used, for example, if the tumor was very large or found to be invasive (spreading). Because the cure rate for ductal cancer in situ is almost 100 percent with mastectomy alone (without follow-up radiation or chemotherapy), some women choose this route over breast conservation.

In any of these options surgeons may remove some lymph nodes from under the arm to make sure there has been no spread (metastasis) of the cancer. Such a spread is unlikely in this type of cancer.

LOBULAR CANCER IN SITU (from the Latin "in place")
Tis, NO, MO

There is some controversy about how to treat this very early cancer, which some regard as pre-cancerous. This cancer is totally encapsulated; i.e., it hasn't spread into the surrounding tissues, but even though it is contained, it does carry a greater risk of later developing into invasive cancer in both breasts. One of the problems with lobular cancer in situ is that there might not be an actual "lump," caused by the body forming hard fibroid tissue around the cancer cells. Instead, the lobular cells fan out and the only sign of the cancer may be a little thickening. The lack of an actual tumor means surgeons may have a harder time making sure all the cells are caught.

Treatment options include a biopsy to remove the tumor, followed by regular exams and mammograms to make sure it doesn't redevelop, or surgery (mastectomy) to remove one or both breasts.

The surgeon may also remove some lymph nodes from under the arm to make sure the cancer hasn't spread.

STAGE I BREAST CANCER
T1, NO, MO

This is very early breast cancer and, with good prognostic factors, has a five-year survival rate of over 90 percent!

In Stage I breast cancer the tumor is less than an inch in size (2 centimeters) and the cancer has not spread to the lymph nodes under the arm.

Possible treatments include a lumpectomy followed by radiation therapy, a partial mastectomy (removal of part of the breast) with follow-up radiation, total mastectomy (removal of the breast) or modified radical mastectomy (removal of the lining over the chest muscles (modified radical mastectomy). In all these cases some lymph nodes under the arm are also removed to make sure the cancer hasn't spread.

In many cases doctors will also recommend follow-up chemotherapy drugs and/or hormonal drugs such as tamoxifen. Research has shown that, even in women with no lymph node involvement, there is a 30 percent chance of the cancer recurring. Chemotherapy and tamoxifen can improve these odds.

STAGE II BREAST CANCER

Stage II breast cancer is divided into IIA and IIB. Stage II is also considered "early" breast cancer, although the survival and recurrence odds are not quite as good. Still, the five-year survival rate is well over 70 percent and considerably higher with follow-up treatments of chemotherapy and/or tamoxifen.

Stage IIA
TO, N1, MO or T1, N1, MO, or T2, NO, MO
- The cancer is less than an inch (2 centimeters) in size but has spread to the lymph nodes under the arm (TO or T1, N1, MO).
- The cancer is between about an inch and two inches in size (2 to 5 centimeters) but has not spread to the lymph nodes. (T2, NO, MO).

Stage IIB
T3, NO, MO or T2, N1, MO
- The cancer is larger than 2 inches (5 centimeters) but hasn't spread to the lymph nodes (T3, N0, M0).
- The cancer is an inch to two inches in size (2 to 5 centimeters) and has spread to the lymph nodes (T2, N1, MO).

Possible treatments for Stage II breast cancer include lumpectomy followed by radiation therapy, or removal of part of the breast (partial mastectomy) followed by radiation, or total or modified radical mastectomy (removal of the whole breast or the breast and the lining of the chest muscles). In all cases the surgeon will also remove some lymph nodes from under the arm. In very rare cases, the surgeon may perform a radical mastectomy (removal of the breast, the chest muscles, and the lymph nodes under the arm).

In some cases, radiation therapy may follow a mastectomy, but this procedure is unusual unless there are many lymph nodes involved.

With Stage II cancer, you will probably receive follow-up treatments, either chemotherapy (especially if you are premenopausal) or the hormone tamoxifen (especially if you are postmenopausal and/or if your tumor is estrogen-receptive-positive). More about these treatments in later chapters. Some patients also receive radiation treatment to the chest to reduce the possibility of recurrence.

If the Stage II cancer is very aggressive or advanced, doctors may apply more drastic measures, such as using even more powerful chemotherapy combinations. The Adjuvant Chemotherapy, Clinical Trials, and Recurrence chapters explain some of these procedures.

STAGE IIIA BREAST CANCER
TO-3, N2, MO
Stage IIIA breast cancer is diagnosed if:
- The tumor is 2 inches (5 centimeters) or smaller but has spread to the lymph nodes, and those nodes have grown into each other or into the chest wall or skin but can be operated on.
- The tumor is larger than two inches (5 centimeters) and has spread to the lymph nodes under the arm.

Treatment for this stage is more drastic because the cancer is larger or it has started to spread beyond the lymph nodes under the arm. In almost all cases, a modified radical mastectomy (removal of the breast and the lining of the chest muscles) will be performed. Some or all of the lymph nodes under the arm are removed. In some cases the patient will even will receive radiation and/or chemotherapy before the operation to reduce tumor size and spread.

The alternate treatment is a radical mastectomy, in which the surgeon removes the breast, the chest muscles and all of the lymph nodes under the arm, but such a procedure isn't used much these days.

Follow-up treatment is imperative here, and the Stage IIIA patient will receive radiation treatments and chemotherapy and/or tamoxifen. There are many clinical trials underfoot to test new drugs to fight this stage of cancer.

STAGE IIIB BREAST CANCER
(Any T, N3, MO, or T4, any N, MO
(May also include Inflammatory Breast Cancer)

This stage cannot be cured or put in remission by being operated on, although the patient may receive a mastectomy following radiation therapy. Tumor size doesn't matter with this type of cancer because it has already spread. Stage IIIB is indicated when:

• The cancer has spread to areas near the breast such as the chest wall, the ribs, or the chest muscles, or

• The cancer has spread to the lymph nodes above or below the collarbone.

After the original biopsy, the treatment for Stage IIIB would probably include radiation to the breast and the lymph nodes, with a mastectomy (removal of the breast) done after the radiation treatments. Chemotherapy and/or hormonal drugs such as tamoxifen may be given before or after radiation and surgery. New treatments are being tested and include drug combinations, biological therapies involving the immune system, and bone marrow transplantation. (A bone marrow transplant means the bone marrow is either replaced, or the patient's own marrow is removed, "cleaned," and reused.)

STAGE IV
Any T, Any N, M1
At this stage, breast cancer has spread (metastasized) to other parts of the body such as the bones, brain, liver, or lungs.

Treatment options include a biopsy followed by radiation therapy and then a mastectomy (removal of the breast) and chemotherapy and/or hormonal therapy such as tamoxifen. Sometimes patients receive a bone marrow transplantation in which high doses of chemotherapy are given to shrink any tumors; then marrow (or donated marrow) taken from the bone, is frozen and replaced when drug therapy is completed. Other treatments, sometimes available in clinical trials, include revving up the immune system to fight the cancer, and new chemotherapies and/or hormonal drugs, including taxol. (More about this in the chapter on Recurrence.)

INFLAMMATORY BREAST CANCER
Because of its aggressive nature, treatment for this cancer is similar to those given for Stage IIIB or Stage IV.

CANCERS OF THE NIPPLE
These cancers are generally treated with radiation or surgery with follow-up treatments dependent on any cancer spread.

AND NOW. . .
So now you have been diagnosed, and you know what kind of cancer you're dealing with. It's time to detail some of the treatment options available for your type and stage of cancer.

5. SURGERY: THE FIRST LINE OF TREATMENT

I
f you are reading this book and have been diagnosed with breast cancer, the chances are good that you will have some sort of surgery. Why? Because the first thing your doctors want to do is to get rid of the known cancer, and in the disease's early stages (in situ, I and II), that usually means getting rid of it through surgery. As oncologist Sandra Swain puts it, "You take out the cancer and then treat the system."[42]

SURGICAL CHOICES: ALTERNATIVES TO MASTECTOMY

The "old" surgical treatment was always a mastectomy (removal of the breast), and often the form of that "old" treatment was the "Halsted," a truly radical and disfiguring type of surgery. Not only was the breast removed but the chest muscles, the fat under the skin around the breast, and all the lymph nodes and fat from under the arm as well.

Today the Halsted is seldom performed, and there is a good chance your breast can be saved. For one thing, cancers are now being found at an earlier stage, thanks to mammography. For another, the medical profession finally agreed with what women such as Betty Rollin and Rose Kushner had been arguing: In many cases, breast cancer could be treated by removing the tumor and surrounding tissue -- but conserving the breast -- and then following up with radiation therapy.

Part of the problem was that doctors were waiting for the results of American research supporting breast conservation surgery (BCS). These studies had to be controlled clinical trials, the "gold standard" of such research. Then, in 1985, the results of such a trial were released: This landmark study, part of the National Surgical Adjuvant Breast & Bowel Project (NSABP), showed that removal of part of the breast (lumpectomy or quadrantectomy) followed by radiation (a treatment program called Breast Conservation Therapy or BCT) was as effective as mastectomy in many cases of early breast cancer. At last there was a gold standard!

But was it fool's gold? Nine years later, the *Chicago Tribune* reported that this large 1985 study contained falsified and/or irregular data from some of the participating treatment centers, including one in Los Angeles, California, and two in Montreal, Canada. Alarmed women throughout the country wondered if their lumpectomy/radiation treatment had really been proved to be as effective as mastectomy in many cases of early breast cancer.

In the end, however, the National Cancer Institute, as well as others in the medical community, concluded that the final results of the NSABP trial had not been changed by the flaws found. One other outcome was the departure, under some duress, of the head of the NSABP study, Dr. Bernard Fisher, for many years a towering figure in the world of clinical trials.

Numerous other studies have since shown the effectiveness of breast conservation with follow-up radiation. The results of a California study, published in 1994 in the *Journal of the American Medical Association* soon after the hullabaloo over the 1985 trial, confirmed the effectiveness of lumpectomy and radiation.

This study, by the way, also showed that patients having surgery in large community hospitals had a much higher five-year survival rate than those treated in smaller hospitals. Patients treated in health maintenance organization (HMO) hospitals had the poorest five-year survival rates for localized breast cancer, regardless of the hospital's size. (HMOs were improving towards the end of the study, and patients whose cancer had spread to the lymph nodes had survival rates similar to those for women treated in "regular" small hospitals.)

Teaching hospitals also performed a much greater percentage of breast conservation operations.[43]

Why? Dr. Arthur E. Baue, a distinguished surgeon with the St. Louis Health Sciences Center, speculated on possible answers in an editorial in the same issue of the magazine. Dr. Baue pointed out that younger patients may seek teaching hospitals, and that older surgeons elsewhere may not accept the validity of breast-conservation studies, or "they may be set in their ways."

Dr. Baue also wrote that, "Some male surgeons may not understand that women value their breasts as part of their person, not because of vanity or sexuality....There is a growing number of women surgeons specializing in the treatment of breast cancer who are successful because they understand their patients."[44]

Evidence is mounting that, even with the smallest of ductal cancers in situ, radiation therapy will decrease the possibility of such a recurrence within the breast. The same is true for women with early Stage I cancers. So, if you are going to go with the lumpectomy/segmental route, you should probably also include radiation.

It's easy to decide to go with a lumpectomy and then put off any radiation therapy, but, as Dr. Diana Farrow of the Fred Hutchinson Cancer Center emphasized at an NCI workshop, "Getting radiation should be part of the initial decision process."[45] In other words, if you consider lumpectomy -- even if you have what your surgeon calls "clean margins" around your tumor -- you *must* also consider radiation therapy as part of your treatment, unless your physicians explain why it is not necessary in your case.

There are possible exceptions. Young women under 40 may be slightly more at risk for developing cancer in their other breast after radiation. Older women well into menopause who have a quadrantectomy (removal of a quarter of the breast) may have tissue changes that could reduce the necessity for radiation. But for the most part, you must think radiation when you think lumpectomy or other breast conservation surgery. Please read chapter on Radiation.

MASTECTOMY: TRAUMA OR CHOICE?

Even today, not every woman can have lumpectomy/radiation, either because of the size or location of the tumor or because of cancer spread within the breast. And not all women *want* to keep their breasts. In 1992 Dr. Swain told a group of cancer survivors that half of her patients at the Lombardi Cancer Research Center in Washington, D.C., still chose mastectomy. One reason might be that, with ductal cancer in situ or small invasive cancers, the survival rate with a mastectomy is close to 100 percent. And radiation is not without its own side effects, not to mention the expense and time-consuming nature of the treatments.

Although many early breast cancers are eligible to be treated with lumpectomy and radiation (including small cancers or a single tumor of up to two inches in diameter), many women still opt for a mastectomy because they are scared of cancer later reappearing in that breast. Then there are the problems of getting regular radiation therapy; in some parts of the country it isn't possible to find a hospital offering such treatments.

The trauma of the loss of a breast became "public" when artist Matuschka posed half "topless," the half showing the scars from her mastectomy, on the cover of the August 15, 1993, issue of *The New York Times Magazine*. The reaction was powerful, pro and con, but it was a watershed moment for mastectomy, perhaps, "opening up a door of freedom" as Matuschka herself put it. "This is my natural look" was Matuschka's response when asked by a tv interviewer why she was displaying her mastectomy, both in print and in her art.[46]

Facing the after-effects of a mastectomy, including the scar, is, however, one of the most traumatic moments a woman with breast cancer faces, even though today's mastectomy is much less disfiguring than the old "Halsted." Although they can usually have reconstruction down the road, many women eventually accept their breast loss, and some are even glad to get rid of something they hold responsible for their illness.

It is psychologically important, however, to get a prosthesis and appropriate bras as soon as possible. Usually, these are medically deductible, and if your remaining breast is large, they will also give you the body balance you need. (See Coping chapter.)

If you are thinking about a mastectomy, or your tumor is quite large or in a place (such as behind the nipple) that makes lumpectomy or segmental surgery difficult and a mastectomy necessary, you owe it to yourself to look into reconstruction before you make any final decisions. You may even be a candidate for immediate reconstruction. (See chapter on Reconstruction.)

MAKING SURGERY EASIER

There are a couple of things all women should do before contemplating any surgery: First, stop smoking. These "coffin nails" are hard on the heart and lungs, and smokers have two to three times the number of problems with healing as non-smokers, along with higher levels of lung and heart complications. If you can't give up smoking for good, at least try going without cigarettes for a couple of weeks or several days before surgery.

"After 12 to 72 hours of not smoking most of the short-term harmful effects that nicotine and carbon monoxide have on the heart clear," Dr. Jay Siwek, a Washington, D.C. family physician and columnist, advised in *The Washington Post Health* Magazine.[47] He also suggested trying to stop without a nicotine patch, which has its own poisons to offer surgical patients.

You should also cut out aspirin or other blood-thinning drugs (unless your doctor advises otherwise) before any surgery. If you are premenopausal and decide on a mastectomy, schedule it towards the last part of your menstrual cycle. Odd as this may seem, there is evidence that having this surgery at the end instead of the beginning of the cycle reduces the possibility of recurrence.

The results of a Milan, Italy, study, published in *The Lancet*,[48] showed premenopausal patients (with positive lymph nodes) having breast cancer surgery during the last 14 days of their menstrual cycle had a five-year relapse-free survival rate of 75.5%, compared with a rate of 63.3% among those operated on during the first 14 days of the cycle.

Before you decide on any treatment, know that you will have to remain flexible. If, for example, your surgery shows up even one positive lymph node, you will probably have to have chemotherapy and/or tamoxifen in addition to any radiation treatment already scheduled.

TYPES OF SURGERY

Biopsy

In some cases, if the surgeon removed all the cancer plus some additional tissue around it during the original biopsy, and the cancer was totally contained (in situ), no further surgery may be needed. Later, however, the surgeon may remove some of the lymph nodes from under the arm to check whether the cancer has spread. Removal of the nodes requires anesthesia.

Lumpectomy

In a lumpectomy the surgeon removes the breast tumor plus some normal tissue all around it. At the same time he or she may remove some of the axillary lymph nodes. General anesthesia is required for this operation.

Breast Surgery

Many surgeons also remove some or all of the underarm lymph nodes to check for possible spread of cancer. (See Modified radical mastectomy illustration)

In *lumpectomy*, the surgeon removes just the breast lump and a margin of normal tissue around it.

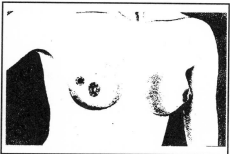

Lumpectomy

In total (simple) mastectomy, the whole breast is removed.

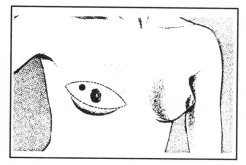

Total mastectomy

In partial (segmental) mastectomy, the tumor, some of the normal breasttissue around it, and the lining over the chest muscles below the tumor are removed.

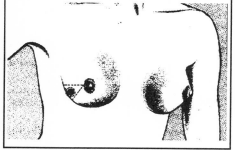

Partial mastectomy

This procedure removes the breast, the underarm lymph nodes, and the lining over the chest muscle.

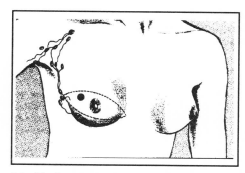

Modified radical mastectomy

National Cancer Institute

Quadrantectomy or Segmental Mastectomy

The surgeon takes out the tumor plus some normal tissue and the lining over the chest muscles near the tumor. Some or all of the lymph nodes are removed. General anesthesia is required and the cosmetic results may not be quite as good as for a lumpectomy but may assure that the "margins" are completely clear around where the tumor was.

"Simple" or Total Mastectomy

All the breast tissue is removed as well as some or all lymph nodes under the arm, so it's not so "simple," despite the name. The incision and resulting scar will probably run across your chest.

Modified Radical Mastectomy

This is the type of mastectomy usually performed today. The surgeon removes all of the breast tissue, the lining over the chest muscles and some or all of the lymph nodes under the arm. Occasionally some of the chest muscles are removed as well.

The incision -- and later the scar -- will usually run diagonally across your chest.

Radical Mastectomy (also known as the "Halsted Mastectomy")

Once the most common operation for breast cancer, this drastic procedure is now almost never performed. In this operation the entire breast was removed, as well as the chest muscles and all of the lymph nodes under the arm. The surgery sometimes resulted in swelling of the arm and loss of some shoulder muscle as well as leaving the patient with a hollow chest area.

WHAT TO EXPECT BEFORE SURGERY

Most hospitals will require various tests before surgery. These include a chest x-ray, an EKG (electrocardiogram) to make sure your heart is functioning properly, blood tests, and a urinalysis to check your kidney functions.

You will also be tested for your blood type in case a transfusion is needed. With testing procedures and screening in use today, blood is fairly free of the viruses that cause AIDS and hepatitis, but, if your surgeon thinks you may need a transfusion, consider giving your own blood ahead of time. It's even safer.

Most hospitals used to have patients check in the day before surgery, but now they are often admitted early on the actual day of surgery. Insurance companies prefer this route since it saves on costs.

You will probably be told not to eat or drink anything after the midnight preceding surgery. This is a very important rule to follow. If you ignore it, you invite disaster -- you may even try to throw up in the middle of the operation. If vomit is aspirated into the lungs they can be damaged -- a complication you don't need!

Some hospitals allow, or even prefer, for you to pre-register. This enables you to fill out all the various forms a day or more before the operation. This paperwork includes consent forms (for the operation), medical history (allergies, etc.), information for the anesthesiologist, insurance status, etc. You will also undergo any necessary blood tests, EKGs, chest x-rays, etc.

You will either be assigned a room before surgery or go to a staging (in-patient) area where you'll change into your hospital garb. Your outfit will probably include tight stockings on your legs. These stockings help prevent blood clots from forming. Sometimes you may be put in "stockings" that actually "pump" your legs during, and even after, surgery. Your surgeon and the anesthesiologist may visit you before the surgery.

Once you're in the operating room, the anesthesiologist will insert an intravenous (IV) needle into a vein in your hand or arm for administering "food" (glucose or a similar substance), anesthesia, painkillers, antibiotics, or even a transfusion if necessary. A monitor will be attached to check your heartbeat and blood pressure during the operation.

Other people in the operating room will check your lungs, heart, and other vital signs and cover your head with a shower-like cap. Usually, you'll know when the anesthesia is starting and then. . . you're asleep.

WHAT TO EXPECT AFTER SURGERY

If you have major surgery (lymph node removal, quadrantectomy, mastectomy, reconstruction), you will probably be taken to a nearby recovery room where your post-operative condition can be carefully monitored. (Sometimes patients are taken to the intensive care unit for monitoring.)

When you awaken from the anesthesia, you may feel very groggy and not want to do anything but sleep. You will still have an intravenous line attached to your arm or wrist which will be "feeding" you -- giving you the nourishment you need and perhaps even antibiotics and pain killers. The feeder line for the IV is attached to a pole and you will find it awkward but not impossible to move around while you are attached to this pole.

Your goal -- to go to sleep -- may be counter to the objectives of the nurses and other aides around you. They will be taking your blood pressure and temperature while urging you to try a first trip to the bathroom. If you've been under anesthesia for a lengthy period of time, you will probably also be given a plastic tube with instructions for inhaling and exhaling to improve your lung capacity. (Anesthesia is not particularly good for the lungs and nobody wants yours to fill up with fluid, a condition that can develop into a form of pneumonia.) You may be nagged to do this and that, all for good purpose. Your chores are important and you should end up doing them even if you don't want to.

If you had lymph node surgery and/or a mastectomy, you will also have a drain under your arm to take away fluids that accumulate. You will probably stay in the hospital until the drainage tube can be removed for good. In fact, you should talk to your surgeon about this ahead of time so that he or she can persuade your insurance company or HMO to allow you to stay. Your insurance company, of course, wants you out of the hospital as soon as possible!

Your underarm area and that of the mastectomy/segmental incision will have been bandaged. Areas of the chest and arm and underarm may feel numb. If you have had a mastectomy or immediate reconstruction, you may have contractions of the chest muscles. These contractions can cause considerable pain that is easily controlled, however, by painkillers.

With lymph node dissection, you may also find you can't lift your arm much. With your doctor's permission, the Reach to Recovery people can visit you. This is a volunteer program sponsored by the American Cancer Society. The "Reach" in the program is talking about your arm just as much as about your ultimate recovery. The volunteer, who has usually had breast cancer herself, will provide a sympathetic ear as well as exercise tips and, if you've had a mastectomy without reconstruction, a temporary breast form (prosthesis) and bra, as well as information about your recovery. Arm and shoulder exercises are very important, but you must have your surgeon's permission to start them. (See chapters on lymph node surgery and coping.)

Except for arm and shoulder stiffness, recovery from lumpectomy, lymph node dissection, modified radical mastectomy, and even immediate implant reconstruction, is amazingly quick, because, as surgeons point out, the body cavity has not been invaded. Patients undergoing a hysterectomy, for example, have a much longer recovery period. Unless you have the more drastic "tissue flap" type of reconstruction, you should be able to resume many of your normal activities within a couple of weeks or so. You may feel tired for a while longer, and your arm will need time to heal and regain dexterity. Even so, I gave a party for 85 people at my house three weeks after my operation (mastectomy with immediate reconstruction).

Tips: Massage your scars with aloe, cocoa butter or fluid from Vitamin E capsules. Keep practicing deep breathing and don't forget those arm exercises, once you're allowed to begin them. (If you have had reconstructive surgery, you'll have additional "chores," but it's worth it.)

6. LYMPH NODE SURGERY
AND YOUR ARM

Remember those glands around on your neck that get tender when you have a bad sore throat? They are part of the lymph system, a first line of defense against such infection. The same thing is true of the lymph nodes under your arm -- they are a first line of defense against breast cancer spread. Lymph nodes near the breast include those under the arm and behind the chest wall. Tiny (micrometastatic) breast cancer cells can find their way into these nodes and from there spread to other parts of your body.

So, unless your cancer is completely contained (in situ), your surgeon will take out some or all of the 30 to 60 lymph nodes under your arm (axillary node dissection) for biopsy. Nowadays surgeons are generally inclined to take fewer -- more like 10. There are three levels of nodes, and each node is about the size of a kidney bean. Surgeons can't tell exactly how many they are taking out because the nodes are encased in fat pads. Even today, however, you'll find surgeons who won't discuss the matter and won't even tell you the number of nodes they removed!

Ask a surgeon why this whole procedure is necessary and he or she will explain, as surgeon James Wolcott does, that this is a major diagnostic tool. "We need to take lymph nodes," he says firmly. In fact, the staging of breast cancer (I, IIA, IIB, etc.) for treatment is based in part on the status of lymph nodes. Until researchers develop another way to determine whether cancer cells have spread to the lymph nodes, whatever surgery you select will, in many cases, include at least a lymph node "sampling."

Like the circulation system for blood, the lymph system has vessels (lymphatics). They drain a watery fluid, lymph, back into the blood stream. These vessels are connected by the lymph nodes, which contain white blood cells to trap any invaders and fight infection. A surgeon can either take a sampling or may remove all of the nodes under your arm for biopsy.

If none of the lymph nodes shows cancer, the patient is "node negative" and the odds are better that she will remain cancer-free. Likewise, the odds for a patient with one to three positive lymph nodes are better than those for someone with four or more. Chances are that any patient with any lymph nodes with cancer cells will have additional (adjuvant) treatment such as chemotherapy. If there are a lot of lymph nodes involved, doctors may prescribe more drastic procedures such as radiation to the area or even a bone marrow transplant.

WHAT THEY DON'T TELL YOU

Removing the lymph nodes under your arm is a big deal -- even taking a sampling of the nodes involves cutting through muscle and nerves. The operation itself takes at least an hour, and considerably longer if all nodes are removed. Although lymph node removal is a major way to determine the status of your breast cancer, it sometimes can make the arm painful, weak, or even swollen. And there may be lifelong complications. Chances are you will already have had a biopsy as well as pathological information about your cancer before you have any lymph node surgery. So, unless there is reason to suspect that your cancer is very aggressive or advanced, you may want to ask for -- make that demand -- a lymph node sampling; i.e., removal of some of the lower nodes (axillary tail) nearest the breast.

There is a new treatment on the horizon: Surgeons in California have developed a dye-mapping procedure which may determine if cancer has spread to lymph nodes. If the procedure shows no spread, the patient won't have to have her nodes removed.

In the meantime, here are the complications you may face, *even if all the nodes removed are cancer-free*, especially with extensive lymph node surgery.

COMPLICATION NUMBER I: *Numbness, Tingling, Pain*

After the operation your underarm area will be bandaged and you will have a tube under your arm to drain away any excess fluid. You may experience swelling, numbness, pain, and tightening of your arm, shoulder and even the chest area. There may be a big "bump" under your arm which will gradually disappear. Unless you had a mastectomy and the lymph nodes were removed through the same area, you will have stitches under your arm. These will be taken out in a week or so.

The numbness is caused by nerve damage and may last a long time, some of it perhaps forever. Generally, feeling will come back gradually, from back to front, and you may experience some itching or pain as this happens.

Lymph node removal can also cause a dart-like pain that can run down your arm. Pain, as well as numbness, can continue for a long time, sometimes forever. Some people also experience nagging headaches.

After the operation you should be on the lookout for inflammation and tenderness.

COMPLICATION NUMBER 2: *Restricted Use of Your Arm*

Immediately after your operation, you will be unable -- and you shouldn't try -- to do such things as raising your arm to eye level. But within a couple of days you will have to start exercises to reduce this tightness in your arm and shoulder. If your doctor gives permission for the "Reach to Recovery" volunteers to visit you after your operation, remember that the "reach" not only stands for recovery from cancer but recovery of your *arm*.

If you don't see a Reach to Recovery person, you'll need to get exercises from your doctor, his or her nurse, or a physical therapist. It's critical that you do these exercises to prevent permanent tightening of the muscles.

So, as soon as you have *permission from your doctor*, start exercises to stretch the area. Exercise also helps prevent the formation of scar tissue and adhesions that might otherwise form. Remember, don't start exercising on your own: Wait until your doctor and/or a physical therapist or other experienced professional gives you instructions, and *then do the exercises every day*.

You might check with your doctor about doing these exercises recommended by my friend, physical therapist Ruth Dupree:

1. Bend over from your hips to 90 degrees and do circles with your arm.

2. Still bending, have the arm act as a pendulum and swing it back and forth across the body.

3. Clasp your hands behind your head while you are lying down or sitting in a chair.

4. "Climb" the wall with your arm, letting your fingers "walk" up the wall as far as possible. The first time you do this exercise, mark your highest point with a pencil. This way you can watch your progress, just as you might have done with a "growing chart" as a kid. One day you'll look back and be amazed at your progress!

5. With the help of your other arm, bring the affected arm up over your head as far as you can until you experience a slight discomfort. Then move the arm slightly back and forth. (This is a good exercise to do lying flat on your bed.)

6. Get a broomstick, hold it horizontally with both hands, and move it up and down, and try to get it up over your head.

7. Roll your body back and forth on the bed.

8. To help your lungs recover from your operation, lie on your back and fully exhale and inhale, using your lungs (chest), not your diaphragm.

COMPLICATION NUMBER 3: *Lymphedema (Permanent Swelling)*

Obviously, the more nodes that are removed, the more certain the diagnosis of whether the cancer has spread. But one reason to hang on to as many nodes as possible is that, in a small percentage of cases, the arm's lymphatic system is impaired and you become susceptible to infection and to lymphedema, or swelling of the arm. The lymphatic system guards your arm against infection and removes waste from tissues and the circulatory system. If the lymphatic vessels can't remove the necessary fluid, this excess will cause a buildup of the tissue channels in the arm, meaning less oxygen can get through the system to help battle infection, and the channels become clogged.

If this happens, you can develop lymphedema. This swelling is often permanent, and there is no known cure, although putting the arm in some form of a compression sleeve often helps, as do drugs and isometric exercises. Symptoms of early lymphedema include persistent swelling, usually starting with the hand. The first signs of infection, which can become severe, include rash and itching, followed by inflammation and swelling.

Researchers are looking into ways of curing or preventing lymphedema, such as microsurgery to reconnect the damaged lymph vessels and laser beams to open up existing channels.

Dr. Robert Lerner has established a Complete Decongestive Physiotherapy (CDP) at clinics in New York and New Jersey which promise hope of reducing swelling, according to *Parade Magazine*.[49]

For information write: Lymphedema Services, PC, 360 E. 57th St., Dept P, New York, NY 10022.

Although the chances of swelling and infection in your arm are fairly low (about five percent from lymph node removal as distinguished from 50 percent with radiation treatment of the nodes and 10 percent with a radical mastectomy), you must take special care of your arm for the REST OF YOUR LIFE.

The importance of this was reiterated in the response to a question in *JAMA*'s Q&A section asking if patients needed to observe such precautions as having blood pressure readings and blood samplings taken from the other arm "forever?"

The answer was yes, according to Dr. Donald J. Ferguson of the University of Chicago, because "even a limited and careful dissection of the axillary nodes may damage the lymphatic system of the arm. As a result, the remaining lymphatic vessels are more susceptible to any small infection or other inflammation. Permanent injury may follow even the most trivial injury to the skin," he wrote.[50]

According to the National Cancer Institute, these are among the steps you can take to prevent infection and swelling:

• Be careful to avoid burning your hands and arms when cooking.

• Wear sunscreen and don't get your arm sunburned.

• Make sure all your blood tests, injections, shots, and blood pressure tests are done with your other arm.

• Use an electric razor with a narrow head for removing hair from under your arm.

• Carry heavy packages or handbags on the other arm.

• Wash any cuts as soon as possible and treat them with an antibiotic cream.

• Don't get your cuticles cut; use creams and lotions on them instead.

• Wear protective gloves when gardening or using strong detergents, or any harsh chemicals and abrasive compounds.

• Avoid insect bites and stings by using repellent and not wearing perfume outdoors in the summertime.

● Wear loose jewelry on the affected arm and avoid elastic cuffs on nightgowns and blouses.

Any drastic kind of swelling usually occurs within the first year after the lymph node surgery. Don't forget to call your doctor right away if your arm begins to swell, becomes red, or is hot. While you're waiting to see your physician, put your arm over your head and repeatedly squeeze your fist.

While it is important to take care of your arm, you mustn't treat it as an invalid. Use both your arms equally.

Well, now you know why you should discuss lymph node removal with your surgeon!

7. RECONSTRUCTION

If your physician or surgeon recommends a mastectomy for medical reasons, or if your breast would be too deformed by partial mastectomy and/or radiation, you should consider reconstruction. This procedure enables you to have a breast! In many cases, you can have the reconstruction done at the same time you are having the mastectomy and wake up with cleavage. And, although recovery time may be longer with immediate reconstruction, you are not faced with the emotional trauma of losing a breast.

The major benefit of immediate reconstruction is basically psychological at a time "when a very negative thing is happening to you physically," says plastic surgeon Thomas J. Sanzaro. "It's something positive to focus on," he points out.

Another reason for having immediate reconstruction is that the surgeon will be working with tissue that is unscarred, sparing you a more challenging operation when the surgeon must deal with established scarring. You won't, of course, get away free, since you will still have a mastectomy scar, and other scars if you opt for the more complicated flap type of reconstruction.

In the case of very large breasts, the plastic surgeon may have to reduce the size of the remaining breast in order to achieve a good "match."

And, of course, reconstruction adds to the cost, though your insurance company may pay part of it.

But reconstruction is an option you have. Here's how to explore it:

1. Make an appointment with a plastic surgeon specializing in reconstructive surgery. Ask the surgeon who is doing your breast cancer surgery for a recommendation. He or she may

already work with a plastic surgeon. You should also be sure that the plastic surgeon you consult is a member of the American Society of Plastic and Reconstructive Surgeons, Inc.

At your consultation, the plastic surgeon will tell you if you are a good candidate for reconstruction and what the options are.

2. Ask for a brochure about reconstructive surgery and if the surgeon has photographs of other patients who have had reconstruction.

3. Find out, either through the plastic surgeon or your own friends and relatives, the names of some people who have had the type of surgery you are considering, and get in touch with them. This is no time to be shy, and, besides, most former patients are happy to discuss their surgery. The deciding factor for me, for instance, was a call from a friend of a friend about her implant, which she had found totally satisfactory.

4. You'll also have to decide whether you want immediate or delayed reconstruction and which type; i.e., an implant or a flap.

TYPES OF RECONSTRUCTION

1. IMPLANTS

An implant is the "easiest" -- most straightforward form of reconstruction, both from a surgical and a recovery time point of view. Of course, as oncologist Sandra Swain says, "You never get to nest with these things," but neither do you have the more extensive scarring, expense, and recovery time involved in the more complicated "flap" procedure.

The implant is a soft sac, generally inflated with saline or salt water. Saline and silicone implants both have shells made of a silicone "rubber" substance. Unlike the controversial silicone implant, the saline one is inflated with a salt-water solution at the time of surgery, thus giving the surgeon more leeway in adjusting the size to fit the patient.

IMPLANT PROBLEMS

More than a million women have had either silicone or saline breast implants. Although the great majority are satisfied with their surgery, some women claim that the implants, particularly those filled with silicone, have inflicted damage on their immune systems, resulting in such illnesses as rheumatoid arthritis. In 1992 the U.S. Food and Drug Administration (FDA) banned most use of silicone implants because manufacturers had failed to prove they were safe. The FDA did allow an exception: Cancer patients desiring these implants after mastectomy could still get them by joining a clinical trial program.

Many surgeons had stopped using the silicone implant even before the FDA ban because of potential liability. In late 1993, however, the American Medical Association urged that, until they are proved harmful, silicone implants should be made available for both cosmetic and reconstructive surgery.

In spite of the AMA's endorsement of the implants, in 1994 several manufacturers of silicone implants agreed to pay $4.25 billion over 30 years to women involved in lawsuits. And that amount won't be enough! In 1995 Dow Chemical, once the country's largest supplier of silicone implants, filed for bankruptcy rather than face the threat of innumerable lawsuits.

The controversy continued as studies done by the Mayo Clinic and researchers at the University of Maryland and Harvard University found no association between the implants and the connective-tissue diseases implicated.

Saline implants don't seem to offer the same risks as silicone because the salt water solution dissolves harmlessly in the body if the implant ruptures or leaks, something that occurs in about 1 to 3 percent of these implants over the years. If the implant deflates, it has to be replaced, but the surgeon can generally do this repair job by going through a short segment of the mastectomy scar.

Some women claim that their health has been impaired by saline implants as well, and the U.S. Food and Drug Administration has ordered the makers of saline-filled implants to go through an approval process to assure that these implants are safe. (Saline implants came on the market before FDA began regulating medical "devices" in 1976, but the agency can still require a product to go through an approval process to prove its safety and effectiveness.)

Life being what it is, some studies have since hinted that silicone implants might even be good for you!

For the moment, at least, saline implants remain the only form of implant widely available. The situation would really be difficult if the FDA should decide to take these implants off the market until they went through the approval process or because manufacturers couldn't prove their safety. And our litigation-happy society might end up without *any* implants!

THE IMPLANT PROCEDURE

If you have an implant at the same time as a mastectomy, the plastic surgeon works with the surgeon who does the mastectomy. After the breast tissue and any lymph nodes are removed by the surgeon, the plastic surgeon inserts the implant under the chest muscles through the incision for the mastectomy. This procedure cuts down on the amount of scarring. Having an implant adds an hour or two to the operation time and, consequently, the patient is under anesthesia for a longer period of time.

Psychologically, you won't be thinking that you have lost a breast and wondering if you can get up the courage to look at your scar when the operation is over. Gynecologist and obstetrician Alexander M. Burnett told me about a woman who had had a mastectomy when she was out of the country. When she returned to the USA, she had reconstruction. With her, it made all the difference. "Until I had that done, every time I looked in the mirror, I thought I had cancer," she told him. "Now I know the cancer is gone."

If you have an implant, you can even wake up with a comforting bulge under your gown! And, as mentioned earlier, the surgeon will not have to overcome the mastectomy scar contracture (shortening of muscles or scar tissue) later on. Another possible benefit of implants is that you may be able to have a more complicated "flap" reconstruction procedure at a future date, if the implant reconstruction isn't satisfactory. Remember, too, that Dr. Sanzaro advises that "flap surgery may be contra-indicative in some patients."

If there isn't enough skin to cover the implant at the time you have the mastectomy, you'll need a tissue expander, a device that is inserted under the chest muscle. The expander is then filled with a small amount of saline fluid. A tube, or "port," connects the outside of the body to the implant.

About once a week the surgeon will inject more fluid into the expander so that the skin will gradually expand. In about two to six months there will be enough tissue for the surgeon to remove the expander and insert a permanent implant.

Even if you need a tissue expander, you will know that within a few months you'll have a "breast." You'll have cleavage and you'll look fine in a bra or swimsuit. You won't have to wear a prosthesis (removable artificial breast form) or be fitted for special bras.

Although sometimes the original nipple is saved for reconstruction during a mastectomy, many surgeons feel there is a danger that some microscopic cancer cells might have escaped into it. And sometimes the nipple is too near the tumor itself to be saved.

But if you want a nipple, one can be made for you. Several months after the original operation, the surgeon can concoct a nipple using tissue from the chest over the center of the implant and then create the areola, the pinkish area around the nipple, from the abdomen or by a tattoo procedure.

Tattooing only requires a local anesthetic, and you can even watch!

If you do have immediate implant reconstruction, you will probably remain in the hospital for four or five days, or until the drainage tube is removed. (This tube may also be used for draining from the lymph node area.) You will also be given antibiotics for a week or so and some painkillers. A few activities, such as driving, will be limited for a while. But within two or three weeks, except for strenuous exercise, you should be able to do almost everything you did before.

Almost all body types are suited to implant reconstruction, but quality can vary if the patients are very thin or heavy. Sometimes the size of the opposite breast will have to be adjusted for symmetry.

TAKING CARE OF THE IMPLANT

The doctor will instruct you on how to push your implant down to keep it in place; these things have a tendency to "ride" up when they are first inserted. You will also be asked to massage the area for 10 or 15 minutes a day for several months. This massaging is very important because it helps stretch the muscles and will make the implant and the skin over it softer and more natural and may also help prevent scar tissue from hardening around the implant, a complication known as capsular contracture.

You may want to see a physical therapist during your recovery period. Physical therapist Ruth Dupree advises that patients "need to have their surgeons give them an exercise program or get physical therapy."

POSSIBLE COMPLICATIONS

Part of the surface tissue will be numb, perhaps forever. The implant itself may feel hard at first, and scar tissue (fibrous capsular contraction) can develop around it, affecting the cosmetic appearance of the "breast" and causing pain.

"Simple" implant placement

Latissimus dorsi flap reconstruction

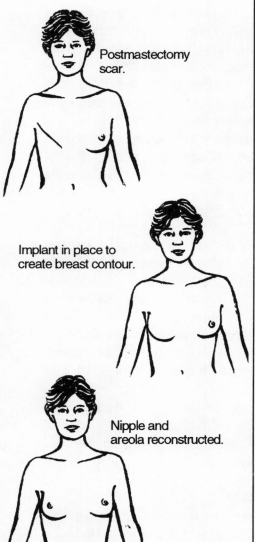

Postmastectomy scar.

Implant in place to create breast contour.

Nipple and areola reconstructed.

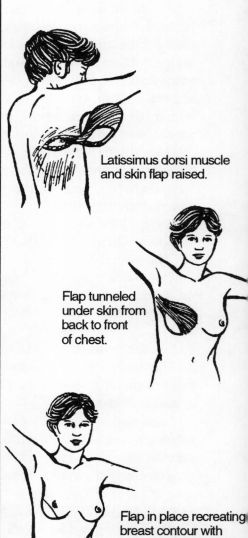

Latissimus dorsi muscle and skin flap raised.

Flap tunneled under skin from back to front of chest.

Flap in place recreating breast contour with reconstructed nipple and areola.

National Cancer Institute

There may be excessive drainage, rejection (less than 2 percent with saline implants), infection, or rupture of the shell of the implant.

Some patients and doctors don't feel a saline implant has quite the natural look and feel of the old silicone one, nor does it seem to move or hang as naturally, and sometimes it has wrinkles or ripples that can be seen at the surface. From an aesthetic point of view, "Most surgeons preferred silicone implants," says Dr. Sanzaro, but he no longer uses them himself. Prices for saline implants have doubled since late 1991, and they were sometimes hard to get. After the FDA's ban on silicone implants, demand for the saline devices exceeded supply for a time; only two companies currently manufacture them. But supplies are okay now.

If you have immediate reconstruction with an implant, you will be under anesthesia longer, and your recuperation period will also be longer. You may experience pain from contractions of the pectoral (chest) muscles which are on top of the implant. This pain can be controlled with pain medication and eventually disappears.

2. TISSUE "FLAPS" OR TRANSFERS

Flaps involve the transfer of tissue from one part of the body to another. Since the tissue is "real" (and tissue from the lower abdomen works especially well), the breast will look and feel real, too. That's the good news. On the other hand, "flap surgery needs serious consideration before being undertaken," says Dr. Sanzaro, although the "results can be very nice."

This operation is much more difficult than the insertion of an implant, and there are greater possibilities for complications as well as more scarring, and often a blood transfusion is required. (Try to donate your own blood ahead of time, if you go this route.)

"Think long convalescence," says Dr. Sanzaro. He also advises younger patients in particular to take a long, hard look at their prognostic factors, including their family history and hormonal receptors before deciding on immediate flap reconstruction. If a younger patient, for instance, has an aggressive tumor, the most important objective is to fight the cancer. The longer recuperation period following flaps may mean any adjuvant chemotherapy is postponed.

Remember, too, that you only have one chance with a flap from the lower abdomen. If you later develop cancer in the other breast, you won't be able to have the same type of flap. (Some women decide to have the other breast removed and have a flap reconstruction on both sides at the same time. This is a serious operation, running 8 to 10 hours.)

On the plus side, the flap operation can be done anytime; for instance, if you decide you don't like your "plain old implant," you can opt for a "flap" at a later date.

Take note: If you are planning to have a flap, it is extremely important that you stop smoking, and take no aspirin or blood thinning medicines before the operation.

TYPES OF FLAPS
1. *Latissimus Dorsi.*

This flap often combines a tissue transport with an implant. The "latissimus dorsi," a flat muscle from the back, along with the skin, is transferred to the chest area. An implant can then be inserted under the flap. There will often be considerable scarring of the back as a result of this procedure.

2. *Transverse Rectus Abdominus (TRAM Flap)*

Dr. Sanzaro says this is the "nicest" of the flaps. This operation moves the rectus abdominus -- the abdominal muscle (one of the two "rectus abdominus" or vertical abdominal muscles) -- and fat and skin from the lower abdomen to the chest area, and the surgeon shapes the tissue into a breast. Because the blood supply comes through the muscle, you could be at risk for tissue loss if there is any problem with the external or venous circulation within the flap.

This procedure also pulls up everything in the abdominal area, giving you the additional benefit of a "tummy tuck" -- and a tummy scar. No implant is usually needed.

You might not be able to get this procedure done if you are very thin or a heavy smoker.

3. *Gluteus*

Tissue is transferred from the gluteus (buttocks) area by microvascular surgery. There may be a good deal of bleeding with this procedure and there is a greater chance of the transferred tissue dying.

RECOVERY TIME

Depending on their complexity, these operations can take from five to 12 hours to perform, and the patient will be in the hospital for several days. A Tram flap will mean five to seven days in the hospital and two to three months of restricted activity. Most patients will require some additional surgery later.

ADVANTAGES AND DISADVANTAGES TO IMMEDIATE FLAP RECONSTRUCTION

On the positive side, psychologically, you won't wake up thinking that you have lost a breast and wonder if you can get up the courage to face the wound. If you have enough tissue to avoid an expander, you'll even wake up with cleavage! The whole procedures will be behind you and you can get on with your life.

Disadvantages to immediate flap reconstruction include a more prolonged recovery. You will be under anesthesia for a longer period of time, making it more difficult to snap back as quickly, and you will probably be in the hospital for several days.

"Rectus abdominus" flap reconstruction

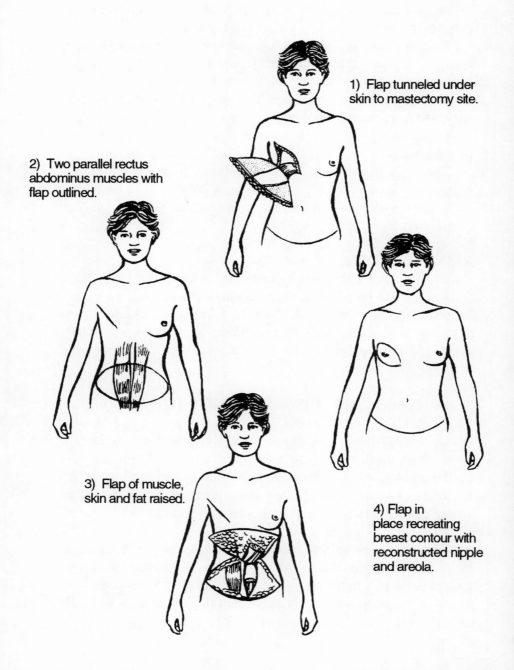

1) Flap tunneled under skin to mastectomy site.

2) Two parallel rectus abdominus muscles with flap outlined.

3) Flap of muscle, skin and fat raised.

4) Flap in place recreating breast contour with reconstructed nipple and areola.

National Cancer Institute

Your body will have to recover from the mastectomy, and the transfer of tissue, as well as any lymph node surgery, and you will have to watch for danger of infection or tissue loss. Any chemotherapy or radiation follow-up treatment may have to be delayed.

ADVANTAGES TO WAITING

If you defer your flap operation, the healing process from the mastectomy, lymph node sampling and any radiation or chemotherapy, can be completed. The flap operation itself will be shorter, and you will have more time to decide exactly what you want. The skin will be more easily movable and elastic if you wait three to six months after the mastectomy. But if you do think you are going to have reconstruction later, you should discuss the possibility with your surgeon and the plastic surgeon before the mastectomy so that the area is better positioned for the reconstruction.

POSSIBLE DISADVANTAGES OF FLAPS

Some of the tissue that was moved may not survive. (This will depend partly on your health and blood supply.) If the stomach muscle (rectus abdominus) has been moved, a hernia or protrusion can develop in a small number of cases. You probably won't have as much strength in your abdominal wall. All of these operations will result in more scarring.

CARING FOR YOUR FLAP

Make sure you follow your doctor's recommendation for oiling and massaging your scars. This massaging may help minimize scarring. Be on the lookout for any infection.

Remember that physical therapy may be very important in helping you regain muscle strength and flexibility. You should discuss treatment with your physician and possibly a physical therapist. If you have had a latissimus muscle flap, for instance, the therapist should know if your physician moved the muscle insertion, Bernard Colan advises in *Advance*, a publication for physical therapists.[51]

In a TRAM flap, the therapist should be told if a mesh material was used to adhere the rectus abdominus area and how much and what muscle was taken during the procedure.

Therapist Ruth Dupree says some patients "don't get instructions from their M.D. but instead do the therapy a friend did after surgery, surgery that might not have been the same kind. This can cause problems."

8. TREATMENT OPTIONS: RADIATION

Mastectomy was *the* standard treatment for breast cancer in America until well into the 1980s! Many in the American medical community resisted change, and it was tough getting the lumpectomy with follow-up radiation procedure introduced into this country. In late 1980 one of my relatives became the *first* breast cancer patient at a major medical facility to receive a lumpectomy and radiation instead of a mastectomy -- and hers was on an experimental basis!

A few months ago I asked oncologist and hematologist James D'Angelo how long lumpectomy/radiation had been a regular procedure at the medical facility where he was practicing at the time.

"Oh, probably six or seven years," was his response. He went on to explain that there was no data (results from a controlled clinical trial) available before then to show that lumpectomy/radiation was as effective as a mastectomy. Another problem was that radiation therapy wasn't as exact as it is today, and some women were left with radiation poisoning of the skin, resulting in permanent blue/black scarring that cannot be helped by plastic surgery or skin grafting.

Now, however, after years of controversy, the results are in: Lumpectomy or quadrantectomy (removal of about a fourth of the breast) *followed by radiation therapy* is as effective as mastectomy in the treatment of early-stage breast cancer. The importance of follow-up radiation is apparent from one of several studies reported in *The New England Journal of Medicine*: Of the 294 patients treated by quadrantectomy and follow-up radiation, only *one* had a local recurrence and no one had a tumor in a new site, compared to 24 with recurrence and four with new tumors in the group of 273 patients treated by quadrantectomy alone![52]   Some studies indicate that adjuvant or "enhancing" radiation can cut the rate of local recurrence from 40 percent down to 10 percent!

The latest studies also show that even patients with very early ductal cancer in situ benefit from this adjuvant radiation. This is particularly true for women who have greater risk factors because of the pathological makeup of their early cancers.

Radiation therapy may be especially important for patients who have infiltrating intraductal carcinoma; even though surgeons do "gross excisions" in order to catch every cancer cell left in the breast, their efforts are not always successful, and such patients have a high risk of local recurrence if they don't have radiation therapy.

Radiation treatment uses high energy x-rays to "zap" -- if you'll excuse the technical term -- any cancer cells that could remain in the breast after surgery. Although these treatments can also be given before or after a mastectomy, radiation's primary use in early breast cancer is after a lumpectomy or quadrantectomy.

In general, today's radiation therapy is administered in much more precise doses, has few side effects, and, in most cases, provides an excellent alternative to the loss of a breast.

Furthermore, clinical trials and other studies indicate that rates of local recurrence and survival are almost identical with for this treatment (BCT or Breast Conservation Therapy) and mastectomy.

SOME CONSIDERATIONS

Radiation, however, is not perfect, and, as my husband, Bill Grigg, a former medical writer who has worked with the

Public Health Service as well as the U.S. Food and Drug Administration, points out: "If you're having drugs such as chemotherapy or tamoxifen, you may have a package insert to read before you start treatment. But there is no 'package insert' available before beginning radiation."

Ask for a brochure about radiation from your doctor as well as any printed materials available at the treatment centers you visit. You can also call the National Cancer Institute's Cancer Information Service (CIS) at 1-800-4-CANCER (or 1-800-422-6237) and ask for any publications which would relate to your upcoming treatment. For more resource centers, see chapter on Coping.

The most surprising side effect of radiation seems to be the high level of fatigue patients may experience during treatment. And this fatigue may linger for several weeks after the procedure is over.

Radiation is very costly; at some high-tech facilities six weeks of treatment can run as much as $16,000. If your insurance only covers part of your treatment, your own bills could run up to $8,000 or even $10,000.

Radiation takes time -- five times weekly over a six-week period. (Some doctors feel this may be too long a duration. Dr. Roy Clark of Princess Margaret Hospital in Ontario, Canada, told an NCI workshop group that four weeks of such treatment was "enough. I can't see any significant difference between the two [time periods]."[53] Even so, this regular treatment can be a regular reminder of breast cancer, a subject you would just as soon not dwell on.)

When combined with certain chemotherapy drugs (melphalen and cyclophosphamide in particular) radiation, particularly to the chest wall or lymph nodes, has in the past increased the possibility of developing leukemia later. The risk is considerably worse with melphalen, especially since lower doses of cyclophosphamide (Cytoxan) are given these days.

The risk of heart problems associated with radiation treatments has declined with the advent of more sophisticated dosage, beaming, and the ability to immobilize the area of the body to be treated. Patients with systemic lupus and some other connective tissue diseases or those with previous radiation for postpartum breast problems should think carefully about entering a radiation therapy program.

Some women experience severe anxiety about the possibility of recurrence of cancer in the breast, even after it has been treated by radiation. These women may be more comfortable opting for a mastectomy.

If cancer does recur in the treated breast, more radiation usually cannot be given to the same tissue area, and in most cases a mastectomy will have to be performed.

If a mastectomy is needed later, radiation-treated skin may not be as responsive to reconstructive surgery.

There is some evidence that younger women treated with radiation may have a greater risk of recurrence of cancer in the other breast as may women with mutations of the BRCA1 gene.

But radiation does give you the option of not losing your breast, and for most people, the side effects will be relatively minimal. Once you've made a decision to go with radiation therapy, your next step is to find the people and the place for your treatments.

FINDING YOUR RADIOLOGIST

Make sure the radiation treatments you get are the best around. Your radiologist should be certified by the American College of Radiology. Ask about the length and type of treatment you will have.

Since you're going to be spending a great deal of time receiving your treatments, it's important that you like both the place and the people where you have them. A good friend of mine, Phyllis Beardsley, who lives in Pennsylvania, made appointments with, and interviewed, the radiation heads at several hospitals before making her choice. Phyllis's visits were "clearly something new" to several of these doctors, "but important for any patient," she reports.

If you don't already have a radiologist and/or hospital you like, it's okay to "shop around." As Phyllis says, "Some people don't seem to know that they do NOT need to have their radiation at the same hospital as the surgery because their surgical oncologist or another doctor may want to keep 'the business' at his or her hospital."

On the other hand, most doctors are not going to recommend anyone they don't respect because any bad results from the radiation will reflect on the referring doctor.

Another reason why it may be important to look around is to find a staff you can be comfortable with. Phyllis felt that one of the pluses of the hospital she selected was the "friendliness and camaraderie of the staff, which I had psyched out in advance. If you don't particularly like the personality of the nurse who does your vital signs during your annual checkup, it's a minor irritation," she says. "But, if the radiation technicians you see 30 or 40 times in five or six weeks are grim, it could make the process doubly depressing."

Feeling comfortable won't assure you of getting the best treatment, however. Ideally, you should try to get the best treatment *and* also be comfortable.

Try to avoid a hospital or clinic that will regularly keep you waiting for a half hour, an hour, or even longer. If you are kept waiting an hour for each of 40 appointments, you are losing another "40-hour week" out of your life in addition to the time the treatments take.

If you don't live in an area with radiation therapy facilities, you need to ask yourself what factor travel time will play in your life. When access to radiation is limited, Dr. Diana Farrow advises women to take this fact into consideration in deciding on treatment options.[54]

RADIATION AND $$$$$$$

Some hospitals and clinics are hesitant to give out cost figures in advance, Phyllis learned, and "make great generous comments about how patients can 'work out an agreeable payment plan,' but when the chips are down and the radiation is over, the finance departments can demand, threaten, and dun you for the full $$$$$$ -- PRONTO."

Patients with no medical insurance, or insurance that pays only part of the bill, should demand at least a ballpark figure in advance of treatment and work out arrangements for payment.

HOW RADIATION IS ADMINISTERED

Your physician will probably discuss your case with a radiologist so that when you see him or her, the radiologist should have already reviewed your x-rays, medical records, and pathology reports. You'll probably also have a physical exam. You may undergo more testing so that the radiologist can determine the dosage of radiation needed, and you will be measured in various ways to determine exactly where the rays will be beamed. The radiologist should explain the procedures to you as well as what you can expect during treatment.

Because radiation must be administered very carefully, and to precisely targeted areas, the technician will mark the exact area of your skin to be treated with indelible ink. Some small permanent dots may be added to pinpoint where the treatment points are. The ink may have to be reapplied because it gradually wears away, but it's important that you leave the ink on while you are under treatment. When you're bathing, be careful not to rub the area and be sure to use only lukewarm water on it.

A specially trained radiation therapist will administer your treatments, which should take only a few minutes. After you change into a gown, you'll be placed on a table and there may be heavy lead "shields" to protect other parts of your body.

You'll be asked to lie very still while the radiation is administered. The radiation may be beamed from more than one angle. In some ways the procedure may prove similar to that you already experienced with chest x-rays or mammograms; that is, you'll be asked to assume various positions and the technician will leave the room to administer the radiation. That's to make sure he or she isn't exposed to stray rays. (After all, the technician does this all the time!)

Generally, you will have these treatments five days a week for four, five or six weeks. One respected addition that many doctors recommend is a "booster" treatment with either radio-active implants near the tumor site or concentrated doses beamed at the tumor area.

Although the daily treatment itself is brief -- and you can receive it as a hospital out-patient or in other medical facilities -- you'll probably find it time-consuming. But aren't all visits to a hospital or medical facility?

Tips: Treat the radiated area carefully. Don't use any creams, deodorants, soaps, etc., without the permission of your doctor and don't scrub the affected skin. Stay away from hot-water bottles, heating pads, and cold compresses. And keep the area out of the sun. Make sure your doctor knows of any medicines you are taking any prescribed by another doctor during treatment. You probably won't be able to shave under your arm or wear nylon.

SIDE EFFECTS

Temporary

The most common side effect is fatigue, which can range from mild to debilitating, and this fatigue can sometimes linger for several months after your treatment is completed. Radiation stresses the body. Some of the fatigue may result from reduced blood counts, but doctors keep careful control of these. (You'll have regular blood tests while you're receiving your treatments.) In the meantime, don't set yourself up for any demanding or challenging projects if you can avoid them. Not only should you take it easy, but you may find it frustrating not to be able to function at top speed. Pamper yourself with extra rest. Phyllis recommends having fun times with understanding friends. Also make sure you maintain a nourishing diet. This is not the time to lose weight!

The skin in the area where you're being treated may turn pink, as though you had a slight sunburn, or it may turn really red, as though you had a severe one, and you may experience some itching or peeling. Later your treated skin may turn darker than the area around it, but this is a temporary condition. Your armpit and/or breast may become tender, or ooze, or even get too dry. Your doctor can give you some excellent medications to treat these conditions.

Two or three weeks after your treatment is over, you may experience a yellowish discharge. Your doctor has medication for this, too.

Long-Term

Your ribs may be slightly weakened and more susceptible to fractures.

The skin texture where you were treated will change, and you should keep this area out of the sun. Make sure you use sun screen when you're wearing a bathing suit.

If you have had the maximum dosage of radiation directed to a particular surface of your body, you cannot have any additional radiotherapy to that area. Your doctor can give you more information on this.

9. TREATMENT OPTIONS: ADJUVANT CHEMOTHERAPY

C hemotherapy! The very word is enough to strike terror into the hearts of prospective patients! Among the most dreaded side effects are hair loss, nausea, mouth sores, weight gain or loss, fatigue, premature menopause, bladder problems, photosensitivity, bands on and/or darkening of fingernails and even fingernail loss.

Yet "adjuvant," or treatment enhancing, chemotherapy is used more and more for patients with early breast cancer. Adjuvant chemo is almost always recommended for pre-menopausal and "peri" (in the middle of) menopausal women who have lymph node involvement. Today it is also often recommended for those with no spread to the lymph nodes under the arm. That is because we now know that 30 percent of patients with no lymph node involvement will still have a recurrence of cancer, but nobody knows who that 30 percent will be. Adjuvant chemotherapy can reduce the percentage of these recurrences.

Unlike radiation/lumpectomy, adjuvant chemotherapy has been used for the last two decades, notes hematologist and oncologist James D'Angelo. "When I first came into practice in 1970, however, chemotherapy was not the standard procedure, even for women with lymph node involvement," he says. It was hard going getting patients to accept the idea of chemotherapy because there was no statistical evidence of its effectiveness.

"Twenty or more years ago, I had a patient with 15 positive lymph nodes," he recalls. "Although it wasn't standard treatment at the time, she accepted chemo and today she is fine."

By the middle and late 1980s, however, the benefits of adjuvant chemotherapy were being noted in various clinical trials in the U.S. and elsewhere. Then, in 1992, a British journal, *The Lancet*, published the results of the Oxford Overview, a study of 75,000 women from 133 clinical trials all over the world. This study indicated that, if treated with adjuvant chemotherapy and/or the hormonal drug tamoxifen, 100,000 *additional* women out of every one million would survive at least 10 years.

Postmenopausal women with positive lymph nodes treated with both adjuvant chemo and tamoxifen increased their survival chances by as much as 50 percent!

SO WHAT IS CHEMOTHERAPY?

Simply put, adjuvant chemotherapy is the use of high potency drugs to kill any microscopic cells that might have survived surgery or radiation. The treatment is systemic; that is, the drugs are sent throughout the system.

Chemo drugs are usually given in combination so that cancer cells not affected by one type of drug may be killed by another. Some researchers are trying other ways of administering these drugs -- using one drug or group of drugs for a shorter, more intensive time period and then following up with the next drug or group of drugs.

Because their job is to destroy any malingering cancer cells, these chemotherapy drugs are very powerful, affecting "good" as well as "bad" cells. Chemo drugs are a little like weed-killers that destroy fast-growing weeds; sure, the weeds are wiped out, but other parts of the lawn might get burned, too. With the chemotherapy patient, the fast-growing "good" cells most apt to be affected include those in the bone marrow, the intestinal tract, the reproductive system, and the roots (follicles) of the hair.

Now for the good news: According to *The Lancet*[55] report, there is evidence that "polychemotherapy" (the use of more than one of these drugs) given for more than one month may provide women with a protective shield against cancer that grows stronger with time and may last for ten years or longer. The trials also showed it was usually unnecessary to give this chemotherapy for more than six months. In the past adjuvant chemo was sometimes given for a year or more! (Patients with recurring cancer may still have longer dosage periods.)

Thanks to some new "helpers" in the chemotherapy field, such as effective anti-nausea medicines and a drug that stimulates the production of white blood cells, more patients are able to finish the full course and dose of their chemotherapy treatments. A recent study, published in *The New England Journal of Medicine*, reiterates the importance of patients receiving a full dose of their chemotherapy regimen ("protocol"). This trial, using three major chemotherapy drugs (cyclophosphamide, doxorubicin, and fluorouracil) showed higher disease-free survival and overall survival for women receiving the full dosage of these drugs than in those taking a reduced amount.[56]

With the aid of new drugs that can help restore the red and white blood cells that are zapped by chemo, "the so called high dose treatment is now the standard treatment," according to Dr. Daniel R. Budman, one of the authors of the study, quoted in *The New York Times*.[57]

And, even though adjuvant chemotherapy isn't a piece of cake, the great majority of patients are able to carry on a relatively normal life during treatment. Most side effects, except chemically induced premature menopause, abate after treatment ends.

HOW CHEMOTHERAPY WORKS

In most cases chemotherapy is given on a daily, weekly or monthly basis, with "rest periods" between treatments to give the body's normal cells a chance to recoup. The drugs may be administered in pill form, by injection or by IV (intravenously into a vein) or IM (injected into a muscle). If you were taking "CMF," for example, you might receive the "C" (cyclo-phosphamide or Cytoxan), the "M" (methotrexate) and the "F" (5-fluorouracil or 5-FU) by IV (intravenously or by IV "push") on two consecutive Mondays. (Sometimes the chemo fluids are "pushed" into the vein so the process doesn't take as long.) Or you might begin taking the "C" (Cytoxan) in pill form for 14 straight days. If your chemotherapy is particularly strong or you have a bad reaction to it, anti-nausea drugs could be added to your IV, or you might be given pills to take orally. Sometimes your doctor may also have you take a steroid, prednisone, in pill form, which can enhance the overall therapy.

After the 14 days on this CMF chemo routine, you would have a 14-day "rest period" before the process started over. This 28-day cycle might be repeated six times in a six-month therapy course.

What do you do during the free period? "I tell my patients to live it up," Alison Martin, a well-known Washington oncologist, told me with a sly grin.

CHEMOTHERAPY AND YOUR BLOOD

If you receive chemo, you'll be given routine blood tests to make sure the chemotherapy is working and that your blood levels are okay. For this reason it's very important to have a lab technician, nurse, or doctor who is good at drawing blood. Remember, if you have had lymph node surgery, regardless of whether any cancer was found in these nodes, do not use the affected arm for chemotherapy administration or blood and other tests. Your other arm will have to take you through the entire chemo treatment.

Pay no attention to the line, "You have small veins; I'm having a hard time finding one I can use." *Everybody* has small veins! If you are really having a hard time with vein problems, ask your doctor about getting a plastic tube that connects to one of the large veins leading to the heart that can be used for drawing blood or for chemotherapy injections.

Chemotherapy affects the immune system, partly because it depresses the body's major disease fighters, the white blood cells.   In fact, before the arrival of a hormonal drug, Neupogen, that helps the depressed bone marrow produce white blood cells, many patients had to have their treatment delayed because of a low white blood count.

"You can't replace white blood cells with transfusions," Chris Hejtmancik, a nurse experienced in chemo administration, told me. When the number of white blood cells goes below a certain level, there is great danger of infection because the body can't fight back.   Doctors call this condition "leukopenia," and before Neupogen, they sometimes had to hospitalize their patients, in isolation wards, no less, to prevent infection.

Now, injections of Neupogen usually mean that treatment can go ahead on schedule. Of course, like everything else in breast cancer treatment, it seems, this drug has its own drawbacks. First, it's not cheap; injections may run as much as two hundred dollars each. And Neupogen injections may increase leukemia risk down the road.

You may also experience a drop in the number of red blood cells which help transport oxygen throughout your body. When this happens, you can get anemic. If the anemia is severe, you may be given a transfusion, or, occasionally, another hormonal drug, Epogen, that stimulates the bone marrow to produce red blood cells.   The more common treatment, however, is a transfusion, says Mrs. Hejtmancik.

If the number of platelets in the blood drops too low, the clotting of your blood may be affected and, if this condition becomes severe, you may need a platelet transfusion.

LIVING WITH TREATMENT (Also see chapter on Coping)

With all chemotherapy regimens, you can expect a certain amount of fatigue. Make sure you get plenty of rest and eat right. Your body needs a balanced diet. Good nourishment is important at this time. Eat lots of green vegetables and carbohydrates. And enjoy meat and mashed potatoes -- in moderation. This is not the time to diet, but, remember, some people gain a lot of weight while on chemo, particularly those who experience a gnawing sensation in their stomachs, produced by excess acid, that is mistaken for hunger.

Many people think food is important to treatment success, but remember, this is *adjuvant* chemotherapy, which is usually given in smaller dosages than that used for serious illnesses, and the amount may not be high enough to require extra food.

Other reasons for weight gain include lack of exercise, administration of steroids (prednisone), and using food for nausea control. People who do gain a lot of weight are faced with another problem when treatment is over -- getting rid of their extra pounds.

On the other hand, if you have trouble eating, try smaller meals on a regular basis. Eat good food, not goodies.

Drink plenty of fluids. Be sure your doctor is aware of all other medicines, vitamins -- even aspirin -- that you are currently taking. These substances may interact with the chemo drugs.

If you work outside the home, try to keep to a normal work schedule. If you are at home, keep your schedule as normal as possible. But don't forget to rest when you're tired.

Don't give up! Tell yourself that, if you drink fluids, you help get the drugs out of your body faster. The effects will still be around, but the kidneys and other organs will function better. Do your chores, go to work. The more you can get your mind off this experience, the better.

During treatment, keep a diary. This will provide an outlet for your emotions and also give you a reference as to how you felt about what was happening during the last treatment cycle, as well as what instructions you were given and when.

Believe it or not, chemotherapy can be a sharing experience that brings you and your spouse or Significant Other closer. You may want to ask your husband or a close friend to come with you to your first chemotherapy treatment. If you are having injections, you'll either sit in a chair or lie down on a bed or examining table. Some of the injected drugs may produce a temporary cold feeling as they feed into the vein. Sometimes chemo is given in a doctor's office; sometimes several patients will receive chemo at the same time in a special area set aside for chemotherapy administration.

You will probably never in your lifetime have so many people fussing over you, especially when, as with most early breast cancer patients, you look, and are, basically healthy! You'll have regular checkups, regular meetings with your doctor, blood tests -- all kinds of care. How could any cancer possibly come back when the patient is so thoroughly monitored?

Be sure, however, to call your doctor anytime you experience fever, chills, or signs of infection. Your immune system is being put through the paces and can't cope as well with everyday bacterial and viral onslaughts.

Even during your "free" periods, your blood counts will be monitored, so you can't get too far away from a medical facility. Don't plan on any big vacations. (Some people do, however, have their oncologist or hospital arrange to have another facility give them treatment if they are going to be away for an extended period of time.)

Some patients actually experience depression *after* their chemotherapy is over. (I did.) Perhaps it's because, after the treatments are over, so is the intensive caring. Or maybe it's because the fighting is over and, now, the patient is back on her own.

All of this care is expensive; the cost before insurance or Medicare can run to $10,000 or even more, depending on where you live and where you are treated.

SOME ADJUVANT CHEMOTHERAPIES

The "big four" of adjuvant chemotherapies are cyclophosphamide (Cytoxan), doxorubicin (Adriamycin), 5-fluorouracil, and methotrexate. Most adjuvant chemo treatment involves a combination of some of these drugs. The most common "combos" are CMF which is cyclophosphamide (Cytoxan), methotrexate and 5-fluorouracil (5-FU); and CAF and FAC, two versions of cyclophosphamide (Cytoxan), doxorubicin (Adriamycin), and 5-fluorouracil. The FAC version uses a higher dosage of Adriamycin.

Doxorubicin (Adriamycin) is the most toxic of these drugs, but in some cases may also be the most effective, particularly with patients having more than three positive lymph nodes, according to *The New England Journal of Medicine*. On the other hand, in its editorial, the *Journal* noted that, "For patients with one or a small number of positive axillary lymph nodes, a doxorubicin-containing regimen *or a full dose of cyclophosphamide, methotrexate, and fluorouracil [CMF] can be appropriate adjuvant treatment.*"[58] (Italics mine). In the same issue, a study showed that doxorubicin (Adriamycin) may also be the drug of choice if the original breast tumor contains the oncogene c-*erb*B-2, which may indicate a more aggressive cancer. There was some indication that patients without this genetic factor responded better to the CMF combination of drugs.[59]

Whatever the regimen your doctor selects, ask him or her about dosage. Although the chemo dose-intensity study, published in *The New England Journal of Medicine* in May 1994, indicated that women had a better prognosis when treated with a full dosage of their chemo protocol, the study also showed that higher dosages, given over a shorter-than-usual period of time, resulted in more life-threatening situations without a "significant increase in either disease-free or overall survival." If your doctor wants you to take on a chemotherapy regimen higher than the standard, ask him or her why. If you are interested, you could also ask about becoming a part of a clinical trial. (See chapter on Clinical Trials.)

If, on the other hand, your doctor wants to give you a smaller dosage than the one appropriate for your age, weight, and other factors, find out why. It's important to get the full, standard treatment, whatever your menopausal status. In the same *New England Journal of Medicine* article about studies of chemo dose-intensity, already mentioned earlier in this chapter, the authors reported that,"...postmenopausal women treated with higher doses of adjuvant chemotherapy had a significantly longer survival than those given lower doses."[60]

Don't try to sweet-talk your doctor into reducing your dosage because of fear of losing your hair (or your lunch). It's your *life* you want to keep!

THE BIG FOUR

Cyclophosphamide (Cytoxan)
This drug is given by intravenous injection (IV) or orally. It sometimes can cause nausea and vomiting, bloody urine (especially if given by IV), hair loss (usually moderate), skin darkening, and lung problems, and can also depress the bone marrow.

What to do: Drink lots of fluids while taking Cytoxan. If you have pills for this drug, take them early in the morning so that the drug will be flushed out of your bladder by the end of the day. Regardless of how you get Cytoxan, don't forget to push those fluids. If you are taking Cytoxan by IV or high dosages of the drug, "You have to drink a lot of fluids to avoid inflammation of the bladder, which can cause blood in the urine," says kidney specialist Dr. Emilio Ramos. With oral doses of the drug, you shouldn't experience problems, but you can help protect your bladder by pushing those fluids.

Methotrexate

This drug can be given by several methods, including IV, IM (intramuscular) and by mouth. Possible side effects include nausea, diarrhea, liver damage, and gastrointestinal and kidney problems. Methotrexate can also cause hair thinning, and photosensitivity (sensitivity to the sun). Your liver will be monitored by blood tests because of occasional abnormalities that develop. These are usually reversible once treatment ends.

What to do: Drink lots of fluids to prevent any kidney damage. Don't drink alcohol without your doctor's permission. Wear sun screen and don't sunbathe! Avoid aspirin as much as possible.

5-Fluorouracil or 5-FU

This drug is administered by IV push or drip. It can sometimes cause nausea, vomiting, diarrhea, loss of appetite, skin darkening (sun sensitivity), hair loss, skin rashes, brittle nails and lines in nails, nail loss (rare), and mouth sores. The vein into which the IV runs may darken, but this is a temporary condition.

What to do: Be careful of the sun. Keep nails soft with good hand creams. Avoid fatty foods.

Doxorubicin (Adriamycin)

This is probably the most potent of the four most "popular" drugs. The good news about Adriamycin is that it seems to increase the time a breast cancer patient remains free of any recurrence of the disease, especially in pre-menopausal women.

It is also extensively used if breast cancer metastasizes. (See Recurrence).

Doxorubicin, or Adriamycin, its trade name, is given intravenously and carefully. The drug can cause painful burns if it leaks out onto the skin during the IV procedure.

Common side effects include severe nausea and vomiting, although these can now be better controlled by anti-nausea drugs administered along with the Adriamycin. Total hair loss is almost a given with this drug, and usually takes place before the end of the second treatment.

Adriamycin's most significant side effect is "cardiac toxicity"; the heart muscle can be weakened if high doses are given. The younger you are, the better the heart tolerates this drug.

Other potential problems include mouth sores, liver damage, and eye problems. It is also normal to experience a change in urine color that lasts one or two days after injection.

What you can do: Be sure to drink extra fluids. Plan to take some time off from work for a day or two after treatment, especially if you experience severe nausea. Before starting treatment, buy a wig. This drug can be rough, but, if you need it, you can handle it! Several of my friends have.

OTHER CHEMO DRUGS

Prednisone

This steroid drug, sometimes given to enhance the effects of other drugs such as Cytoxan, has a bright spot; it can sometimes cause a sense of well-being, which may not be well-founded, but what the heck! Prednisone may also cause stomach problems, and you should be careful about drinking alcoholic beverages with it. Your body needs time to adjust when you go off this medication, and it may affect your blood sugar levels as well. Your face may get rounder and you may experience decreased or blurred vision and skin problems.

Mitomycin (Mutamycin)

Mutamycin is given intravenously and can cause nausea and vomiting, and burning pain if any of the drug leaks out during the IV. Other side effects can include fever, chills, sore throat, decreased urination, shortness of breath, and mouth sores, bone marrow depression, and swelling of feet or lower legs.

Citrovorum Factor (Leucovorin)

This derivative of the vitamin folic acid is sometimes given to patients taking high doses of methotrexate to counteract the effects of that drug on normal cells. This way, methotrexate can be used in combination with 5-fluorouracil (5-FU) but without the toxic Cytoxan.

Vincristine

This potent drug may be used in early breast cancer patients who have a high risk of recurrence. It is sometimes combined with Cytoxan and Adriamycin and is more often used in advanced cancer. Occasionally it is added, along with Prednisone, to the CMF combination (CMFVP).

Side effects can include nausea, hair loss, burning pain if the drug leaks out during administration, fever, chills, sore throat, swelling of feet and lower legs, difficulty in walking, dizziness and double vision, drooping eyelids, depression, numbness, or tingling or pain in fingers and toes.

TIMING OF CHEMOTHERAPY

The Y-ME organization asked Dr. William J. M. Hrushesky, a researcher with the Stratton VA Medical Center, to report if timing the administration of cytoxic chemo drugs to take advantage of biological rhythms could help reduce the drugs' toxicity. Among Dr. Hrushesky's conclusions, reported in the *Y-ME Hotline Newsletter,*[61] were that patients tolerated Adriamycin's effects on the heart and bone marrow better in the morning, partly because heart and bone marrow cells were more "robust" earlier in the day, while 5-FU's effects were better tolerated if the chemo was given close to bedtime.

SIDE EFFECTS

Premature Menopause
One unpleasant side effect of these powerful drugs for "older" younger women may be premature menopause. This means that they have to cope not only with chemo but with the physical and mental effects of menopause. Many women feel a loss of femininity at that time -- no more periods, no more babies, but more facial hair, lots of hot flashes, the possibility of osteoporosis, and depression.

Bleak as it sounds, however, there are a couple of positives about this situation: One is that menopause means a decrease in the production of female hormones, including estrogen, which may affect the development of breast cancer. Recent studies indicate that premenopausal women have a better rate of no recurrence and survival if their ovaries are no longer working. In some cases chemotherapy will produce menopause without the need to physically remove the ovaries or to zap them with radiation.

The other positive news is that the hormonal drug tamoxifen may, in some cases, reduce many menopausal symptoms.

And now there is talk of younger cancer patients later being able to receive hormone replacement therapy, which alleviates menopausal symptoms.

Hair Loss (Also See Chapter on Coping)
Hair loss can be gradual, with more and more hair appearing in a brush or in the tub or shower after shampooing, or it can come out in clumps, or -- brace yourself -- it can fall almost all at once. One cancer patient awakened with so much

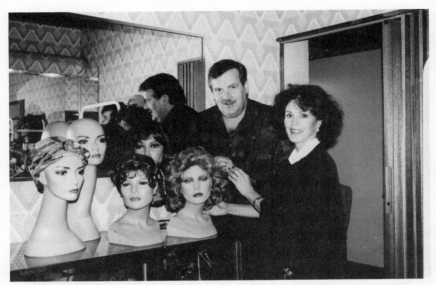

In the "Wig Room" of the Lucien et Eivind Beauty Salon, Eivind Bjerke and Gloria Sansone show some of the items used in the "Look Good...Feel Better" program to help patients cope with losing their hair. Mr. Bjerke's work with cancer patients won him a "Washingtonian of the Year" award from Washingtonian Magazine.

hair in her face that the cornea of her eye was burned. Another reported watching her hairs blow away in a gusty wind. These are horror stories all right, but at least the hair grows back. Sometimes straight hair comes back curly.

Most CMF patients don't lose all their hair. Although most hair loss is experienced during the first two or three treatments, some women have a delayed reaction and have more loss towards the end of the treatment. On the other hand, many people, especially those taking Adriamycin, often see new hair growth before their chemo is finished.

Hair loss may not be automatic with lower doses of Adriamycin and vincristine, according to Doctors Yashar Hirshaut and Peter I. Pressman. In their book, *Breast Cancer/The Complete Guide*,[61] they point out that hair loss may be reduced or prevented if a tourniquet -- a kind of blood pressure cuff -- is used to keep some of these drugs from reaching the scalp. This procedure is particularly effective, they say, in women under sixty.

Another effort to prevent hair loss, putting ice packs on the head before and after treatment, is occasionally used, but its effectiveness is questionable.

Whatever the condition or amount of your hair, keep it away from the chemicals found in most hair colors and permanents. (Most hair colors contain aniline, a chemical you shouldn't mix with chemo.) Health food stores sometimes have color rinses for the hair that contain only "natural" ingredients. Check these, and all other hair color products, with your doctor before using. Some beauty salons offer color rinses that wash out in the next shampoo. You'll also have to be careful with hair sprays containing lacquer, another toxin.

Even if you keep most of your hair, it has been damaged and you may find the texture changed. Hair growth is also very s-l-o-w at this time. Dermatologist John J. Short, M.D., recommends taking a b-vitamin, Biotin, available in health food stores, to strengthen the hair.

For more about hair loss and body image, see chapter on Coping.

Your Skin and Nails

Chemotherapy will affect your skin. You should keep out of the sun and use sunscreen with a sun protector factor (SPF) of at least 15.

Your skin may become drier, and you need to keep it moist. Use moisturizers, but make sure you apply only your own (no borrowing) and also make sure that they are fresh. Chemotherapy patients may have a suppressed immune system and are more susceptible to infection. Keep hands and feet well lubricated to prevent chapping or cracking.

Remember to contact your doctor if you have an allergic reaction to any cosmetic or if you develop any skin infection.

Your nails may become brittle. Keep them short and moisturized. You can use nail polish to disguise any horizontal grooves that develop in the nails, but use only non-acetone based polish remover.

Impossible as it seems, all this will be behind you one of these days!

10. TREATMENT OPTIONS: TAMOXIFEN

For the most part, over the last few decades, the basic treatments for breast cancer have been greatly refined but remain cutting, burning, and poisoning. The truly new treatment is the hormonal drug tamoxifen, now the most widely prescribed cancer drug in the world.

Tamoxifen's debut on the medical stage in the 1960s was a flop. Originally tested as a "morning after" contraceptive pill, it turned out to be a fertility agent. Later, thanks to the efforts of Craig Jordan and others at Northwestern University, tamoxifen was developed as a chemotherapy treatment and first used in advanced breast cancer disease. Since the middle 1980s it has been employed even more extensively as an adjuvant, or enhancing, treatment for women with early Stage I and II breast cancer.

Used in this way, tamoxifen increases survival rates and decreases the probability of breast cancer recurrence, especially in postmenopausal women. In a landmark study (The Oxford Overview) of 75,000 women from 133 clinical trials world-wide, postmenopausal women, with positive lymph nodes and treated with both adjuvant chemotherapy and tamoxifen, increased their survival chances by as much as 50 percent.[63]

The National Cancer Institute recognized the importance of tamoxifen, noting in its journal that, "The worldwide overview of data on 30,000 women with breast cancer in 40 randomized trials of tamoxifen has produced evidence...that tamoxifen, given for an average of 1.8 years, reduced the annual rate of death from all causes by 17%...and reduced disease recurrence by 25%...."[64]

Other studies showed that tamoxifen reduced cancer recurrence by between 25 and 40 percent, increasing survival rates by about 10 percent a year.

Tamoxifen, in fact, looked so good that a new clinical trial was started in 1992 to find out if the drug also would work as a breast cancer preventative in high-risk women. More about that study and its problems later.

What is this "miracle" drug that has been taken by over three *million* women? Basically, tamoxifen (trade name Nolvadex) is an anti-estrogen drug in terms of inhibiting breast cancer growth, but with positive estrogen qualities in terms of helping to prevent osteoporosis (by improving bone density) and heart attacks (by reducing serum cholesterol and by a generalized good effect on blood vessels).

Unlike the drugs ordinarily associated with chemotherapy, tamoxifen doesn't disable or kill cancer cells. Instead it acts as a block to estrogen cell receptors, reducing their ability to multiply. Tamoxifen seems to work particularly well with postmenopausal women whose tumors are estrogen-receptive. In fact, tamoxifen "is the drug of choice" for follow-up (adjuvant) treatment of breast cancer in many if not most post-menopausal women, according to Dr. Barnett S. Kramer of the National Cancer Institute.

The results thus far have been so impressive that tamoxifen is now being given almost routinely as an adjuvant therapy to postmenopausal patients *without* any positive lymph nodes.

One reason tamoxifen seems to work so well in older women is that about 80% of their tumors are estrogen-receptive-positive, while only about 60% of those in younger women are. But this is another area needing more research: One of the findings of the Oxford Overview was that survival and recurrence rates were about the same for younger women given chemotherapy and older women given tamoxifen. Sounds simple enough until you consider that tamoxifen wasn't offered most of the premenopausal women, and the chemotherapy for postmenopausal women was often given in a lower and therefore less effective dosage. This is one of those situations where the kinds of exact comparisons you or I might like are not available.

Originally, tamoxifen was thought to be particularly effective if the cancer was estrogen-receptive, but now it is often recommended for *all* postmenopausal women.

Unlike standard chemotherapy, tamoxifen has few identifiable gross side effects: You don't lose your hair, for example. In some respects this drug has seemed too good to be true; it may also help to prevent osteoporosis and heart attacks. Tamoxifen also often produces a vaginal discharge, decreasing the dryness and subsequent problems with sexual intercourse that many postmenopausal women experience.

Postmenopausal women sometimes find it also eliminates that bugaboo of menopause, the hot flash.

RISK FACTORS

Tamoxifen is, however, a powerful drug and not without its problems. In fact, nobody knows what the long-term effects of tamoxifen are on the body as a whole. Nobody knows how long the drug should be given. Some in the American medical community recommend it be taken for no more than two years; others say it should be given for at least five years. In much of Europe the standard dosage is 40 milligrams a day; in the U.S. the daily dose is half that, or 20 milligrams. Studies seem to point to the lower dosage also being the safer dosage.

Tamoxifen doesn't necessarily work forever, and there have even been cases of women developing tamoxifen-resistant tumors that shrink once the drug is stopped.[65]

Endometrial Cancer
So far, the biggest risk connected with tamoxifen appears to be endometrial cancer -- cancer of the lining (endometrium)

of the womb (uterus). One of the reasons might be that tamoxifen may act much as estrogen does and overstimulate the endometrium. Women taking estrogen replacement therapy after menopause developed more uterine cancer; because of this, the antagonist hormone, progesterone, has been added to most such therapies, and this hormone (trade name Provera) has been added to some tamoxifen protocols.

Studies in Sweden, England, and Denmark had shown some increase in uterine cancer in women taking tamoxifen, but the American bombshell was in late 1993, when new information came to light about a clinical trial supporting the role of tamoxifen in lowering recurrence of early breast cancer. Although preliminary results of this trial, B-14, were released in 1989, information about four later deaths from uterine cancer in trial patients was not reported to the National Cancer Institute until October 1993. In the meantime, women were enrolling in another tamoxifen study, the Breast Cancer Prevention Trial (BCPT), to determine if the drug could prevent breast cancer in high-risk patients. Women joining the BCPT trial, which started in 1992, were asked to sign a consent form that warned them of the increased risk of uterine cancer but also stated no deaths from the disease had been reported in other clinical studies. The consent forms were finally changed in January of 1994.

There was more. Both these clinical trials were part of the National Surgical Adjuvant Breast & Bowel Project (NSABP), a group of studies headquartered in Pittsburgh and supported by the National Cancer Institute and the American Cancer Society. The project was headed by Dr. Bernard Fisher, a revered figure in the world of scientific research.

In 1994 the *Chicago Tribune* reported that falsified data had been included in another landmark NSABP trial, this one showing that lumpectomy/radiation was as effective as mastectomy in breast cancer treatment.

When Dr. Fisher and his associates did release their follow-up report on the "B-14" tamoxifen trial, the incidence of uterine cancer (25 cases) was higher than expected in the group of women taking tamoxifen. Even more surprising was the number of deaths (four); uterine cancer caught in its early stages is highly curable.

Shortly after the publication of the B-14 data, the National Cancer Institute took action. It asked Dr. Fisher and his principal deputy to step aside. (They later resigned.) NCI also suspended all NSABP trials from enrolling new patients, and set up a special monitoring unit "whose sole responsibility will be to assure that the cooperative groups comply with NCI guidelines."[66]

In April 1994 the U.S. Food and Drug Administration announced that a stronger warning about the risk of tamoxifen and uterine cancer would be required in the package inserts sent out with the drug. The manufacturer, Zeneca Pharmaceuticals, sent updated labeling information to 80,000 oncologists and 300,000 other health care professionals. According to *Science*, the magazine of the American Association for the Advancement of Science, ICI Pharmaceutical, Zeneca's parent firm, "had long been pushing for an analysis of tamoxifen's side effects....By July 1993, Zeneca had obtained enough information from NSABP to conclude that patient advisory forms would have to be revised to include stronger warnings."[67]

"Tamoxifen is a valuable treatment for breast cancer, but it is important for women to recognize that there are side effects including an increased risk of cancer of the uterus," FDA Commissioner David A. Kessler stated in announcing the new warnings. He also recommended that women get regular gynecological exams.[68]

In May NCI officials took another step, deciding that the Breast Cancer Prevention Trial could again accept enrollments, in order to bring the study to its full complement of 16,000 (8,000 on tamoxifen, 8,000 on a placebo).

But NCI also stated, "Data from an ongoing treatment trial [B-14]... show that the annual risk of endometrial cancer for a woman taking 20 mg of tamoxifen daily for at least five years is about 2 per 1,000 women per year....Women already enrolled in the BCPT who had not had a hysterectomy" would henceforth "be monitored for endometrial cancer through pelvic examination and aspiration." NCI explained that, "an endometrial aspiration involves removing a small sample of endometrial tissue through a thin tube inserted into the vagina,"[69] a procedure that may be quite painful.

On the minus side of this issue, the women in the trial *don't* have breast cancer, so they are basically healthy women assuming the additional risk of another type of cancer. However, the added risk for uterine cancer from tamoxifen is the same as that for women taking estrogen therapy without progesterone. Why not give progesterone to the women taking tamoxifen in this trial, participants asked at an NCI workshop in November of 1994.

Studies continue. Researchers at Memorial Sloan-Kettering Cancer Center in New York showed that women who took tamoxifen were likely to have an earlier diagnosis of endometrial cancer. Dr. Richard Barakat, lead investigator of the Sloan-Kettering review, suggested that because tamoxifen use can cause vaginal bleeding, it may lead to an earlier diagnosis of endometrial cancer than would have been made if the drug hadn't been taken.[70]

A Netherlands case-control study, reported in *The Lancet* in February 1994 found women taking tamoxifen had a slightly greater risk of endometrial cancer, and that the risk increased with the duration of use. In May 1994 *The Lancet* announced the results of an English study of 111 postmenopausal women. A large percentage of the tamoxifen users developed abnormal and potentially malignant changes in the uterus.[71]

Although an annual biopsy may not be necessary, women using tamoxifen as adjuvant therapy should be aware of uterine cancer risk. Oncologist Sandra Swain recommends that women on tamoxifen therapy see their gynecologist twice a year for an endometrial (lining of the uterus) exam. Instead of a biopsy, you might opt for a vaginal sonogram. This procedure is "highly effective" in detecting any abnormality, according to Dr. Kathy Albain of Loyola University Medical Center.[72] The sonogram procedure can both measure the uterine lining and spot the ovarian cysts that tamoxifen occasionally produces.

If the uterine lining has thickened or if hyperplasia (abnormal tissue) has developed, patients can be given Provera to reverse the process.

Other Risks

A Swedish study of women taking 40 mg of tamoxifen for two to five years showed a six-fold increased risk of endometrial cancer but no additional risk of liver malignancy. These women took double the standard U.S. dosage of 20 mg.[73] Animals have grown liver tumors after high doses of tamoxifen. In another trial two women developed liver cancer out of 931 participants taking 40 mg a day, but no liver cancers have been reported anywhere in trials with women taking 20 mg a day.[74]

Other possible complications are ovarian cysts, colon cancer risk (researchers are still up in the air on this one), eye problems, and blood clots. In younger women tamoxifen may also act as a fertility agent.

Because of the possibility of eye problems, women taking tamoxifen should have regular eye exams (by an ophthalmologist) especially if they have pre-existing eye conditions. The good news is that, in a Greek study trial, most eye problems were reversible once patients went off the drug.

ADMINISTRATION AND SIDE EFFECTS

Tamoxifen (trade name Nolvadex) comes in pill form and is taken twice a day. Drink a full glass of water with each pill.

If you experience any nausea or vomiting, you may be able to reduce your symptoms by taking the drug with food. Try to space the pills evenly by taking one in the morning and one in the evening. If you miss a pill, don't double-dose.

Consult your physician if you have blurred vision, cough or hoarseness, lower back pain, difficulty urinating, shortness of breath or unusual weakness or drowsiness.

The most common side effects of tamoxifen are hot flashes, weight gain, and vaginal discharge. Other and less often noted symptoms can include bone pain (it should go away), pain or swelling in the legs, changes in the menstrual cycle, headaches, vaginal itching, vaginal bleeding or dryness, dry mouth and nostrils, and loss of appetite. These may sound like a lot of symptoms until you remember that every drug has a list of side effects. (Try reading the list of complications and warnings for some familiar antibiotics in the *Physicians' Desk Reference*, a tome describing prescription drugs.) Some women also complain of depression. Tamoxifen may also make you more fertile, so if you are premenopausal, you should take precautions against getting pregnant at this time. Warning: Don't take birth control pills! They contain estrogen, which may be harmful.

Perhaps the most annoying side effect comes from hot flashes, especially in younger women. (In older women tamoxifen may actually help prevent these annoying incidents.) Hot flashes can sometimes be helped by Vitamin E or low-dosage amounts of drugs for reducing high blood pressure and nervous tension such as Clonidine, Bellergal, or Thorazine.

In spite of tamoxifen's drawbacks, Jeff Abrams, M.D., of the NCI's Division of Cancer Treatment, offered these words of encouragement about the drug: "Women who are taking tamoxifen as treatment for breast cancer should be assured of the benefits of the drug in reducing the risk of breast cancer recurrence and in reducing the risk of new breast cancers....the overall survival benefits...far outweigh the risk of other tumors.[75]"

In starting treatment with a strong drug like tamoxifen, it's natural to worry about possible side effects, and you should talk to your doctor about the drug before you begin. Once you start taking tamoxifen, however, make sure that you are suffering from side effects, and not nerves, before you give up on the drug, and by all means talk to your doctor about any symptoms! In a study of tamoxifen and bone density in postmenopausal women, noted in *The New England Journal of Medicine*,[76] a total of nine women dropped out of the test because of side effects. Five of these women were taking tamoxifen and the other four were taking a placebo, an innocuous pill which could not cause any symptoms!

11. OTHER TREATMENT OPTIONS

T here are other, less commonly used treatments for early (Stage I and II) breast cancer. These, too, are part of the battery of first line defenses against recurrence of the disease.

OVARIAN ABLATION (Eliminating Ovarian Function)

The British Imperial Cancer Research Fund "Oxford Overview" of 133 clinical trials involving 75,000 women world-wide, found three of five early breast cancer treatments to be most effective. These three, as published in *The Lancet* in 1992, were tamoxifen, polychemotherapy (more than one chemo given at the same time), and "ovarian ablation," or removal or destruction of the ovaries, in women under 50. Surprisingly, this is an "old" treatment, dating back about 100 years, that has come back into vogue.

In ovarian ablation the ovaries are either removed (oophorectomy), or put out of action with radiation or chemotherapy. The idea behind zapping the ovaries is to cut out the estrogen they produce. In a feature on breast cancer in *The London Sunday Times Magazine*[77] author Peter Martin reported ovarian ablation gives a 10% better chance of survival for premenopausal women than chemotherapy alone. When *The Lancet* published the Oxford Overview (Early Breast Cancer Trialist Collaborative Group) in 1992, it also editorialized that ovarian ablation deserved re-examination:

"It is clearly effective, has continuing benefit, and may be responsible for at least some of the beneficial effects of adjuvant chemotherapy in these patients."[78]

The Lancet also noted that the benefits of this procedure might have the same lasting effect that postmenopausal women taking tamoxifen experienced.

Adjuvant chemotherapy itself may produce early menopause in "older" younger women, those over 40, but the effects are more temporary in younger women. More study of this issue is underway.

One of the American clinical trials in progress is a comparison of two groups of premenopausal node-negative women taking tamoxifen versus those taking tamoxifen and having their ovaries removed (oophorectomy) as well.

Women undergoing any form of ovarian ablation are plunged directly into menopause, with all the unpleasantness of hot flashes, depression, increasing facial hair, bone depletion, and other miseries. And, of course, these women will never be able to have more children.

2. PREOPERATIVE CHEMOTHERAPY OR RADIATION

In some cases, especially when the tumor is exceptionally large, doctors may employ chemotherapy or tamoxifen to shrink the tumor before any surgery. Trials of this procedure in London, Edinburgh and Milan have so far shown excellent results. In the Milan study, of women with very large tumors headed for major surgery, results showed mastectomies were avoided in 91 percent of the cases.[79]

3. PROPHYLACTIC MASTECTOMY

Women with a very high risk of breast cancer or those who have already developed cancer in one breast may opt to have both their breasts removed as a preventative measure. Such mastectomies are usually followed by reconstruction. The TRAM flap may prove particularly effective if both breasts are going to be removed at the same time. (See chapter on Reconstruction.)

4. RADIATION

If a woman has a large tumor and/or many lymph nodes are involved, she may have radiation to the lymph node area and/or the chest wall after a mastectomy to reduce the risk of recurrence.

5. EXPERIMENTAL DRUGS

Clinical trials are constantly underway to test new drugs that may be helpful in the fight against early breast cancer. Researchers are striving to understand the biological makeup of the disease in the hope of developing drugs that can fight its known growth factors. Another area under study is the possibility of inhibiting angiogenesis; that is, the growth of blood vessels necessary for tumor growth. Retinoids (those Vitamin A cousins) and a birth control hormone (Gn-RHA) that can suppress ovulation, are other therapies under study. You'll find more such experimental drugs discussed in the Recurrence and Clinical Trials chapters.

12. GETTING INFORMATION BEFORE YOU MAKE DECISIONS

In the "old" days, when a woman with a suspicious breast lump ended up on the operating table, she didn't know if she would wake up with a breast or not. With the woman still under anesthesia, the surgical team waited while a "frozen section" of the biopsied area was submitted to the pathologist for immediate examination. If the frozen section showed cancer, the surgeon proceeded with a mastectomy.

This practice was still prevalent in the 1970s! Nowadays, however, the biopsied tissue is examined more thoroughly before any decisions are made about treatment for the cancer. You should be a partner with your doctor in the treatment choices open to you.

One reason doctors used to insist on an immediate mastectomy was that they believed that the cancer would spread like crazy if they didn't get it out quickly. Now doctors know that breast cancer, particularly in its earliest stages, is a slow-growing disease, and the medical community has learned that it's okay to wait for several weeks before starting treatment.

This "window" is the time you can use to get any additional information you may need, to get second opinions, to talk to other women who have faced the same issues you must deal with. And the first person on your list to talk to is the doctor who is handling your case. Your physicians may include an oncologist (a doctor who specializes in cancer treatment), a surgeon (who will do your biopsy and any follow-up surgery), a plastic surgeon if you are having reconstruction, and a radiologist if you're having radiation. Your oncologist will probably be your primary doctor.

Some hospitals and/or physicians have programs of "Comprehensive Consultation," where the patient meets with all the doctors who would be involved with her treatment and hears their opinions at the same time. Dr. Julia Rowland of Georgetown University Hospital calls this "one-stop shopping."

Some facilities also have inter-active computer programs where, again, the patient can review various options while sitting at a computer terminal.

Dr. Rowland says doctors recognize several types of patients including the one, often an older woman, who says to her physician, "You decide for me."

The "I demand you do such and so" type is usually a younger and more sophisticated woman, while the over-whelmed patient may say, "I can't decide." She may need some time out to think. The ideal patient is probably some-where in the middle, listening to the recommendations and collaborating with her doctors in the decision-making process. Dr. Rowland also noted that "social support," particularly one's husband but including relatives and friends, "makes a difference."[80]

TALKING WITH YOUR DOCTOR

According to Dr. Rowland, 90 percent of women do want to participate in the decisions about their treatment. Don't be afraid to ask questions. Your *life* depends on the answers! Although patients who pepper their doctors with questions and participate in the decision-making process are sometimes regarded as pests, studies show they often get better faster because they get better care.[81]

Make sure your doctor shares all test results with you. For example, does the final pathology report from the biopsy show favorable or unfavorable prognostic factors: Tumor grade, positive or negative estrogen receptors, DNA analysis (ploidy or aneuploid, high or low S-phase), cathepsin measurement and tumor size. Make sure you know what these and other findings mean so that you can discuss them intelligently with your doctor. All these factors, plus your own feelings, must be considered in decision-making.

Of course you are terrified, and, in that state, may misunderstand or misinterpret, or even forget, what your doctor says, so it's important to have somebody -- your husband or Significant Other, or a close friend or relative -- with you. Ask that person to take notes on what the doctor is saying. You may think you are absorbing every word but, trust me, you aren't. Dr. Rowland calls this the "information gap" that can occur between patient and doctor because of the patient's state of mind. You are under terrific stress and even though you may think you are paying close attention, you may forget more than you remember.

INVOLVING YOUR LOVED ONES

Try to involve your husband or someone else particularly close to you when you are talking to your doctors and getting second opinions. I was surprised (and pleased) when, after listening to the options offered, my husband indicated that he was in favor of the more drastic treatment -- mastectomy -- in my case because it offered the least chance of complications and the best chance of cure. When I told my doctor that I had decided on mastectomy followed by immediate reconstruction, he turned to my husband and asked, "Do you agree?"

"Yes," Bill said. "That's what I've been for all along."

And that's when it finally sank in -- Bill was more interested in my *life* than my breast! And that's what mattered!

SECOND OPINIONS

You may think your doctor is the greatest, but you owe it to yourself to get a second opinion on everything you can, including surgical options, radiation, plastic surgery (reconstruction), etc. This is YOUR LIFE we're talking about.

Sometimes the second opinion may bring you up short because your own doctor may be someone you've known for years. He or she naturally wants to be reassuring. In my own case, I was thinking of the easiest way out after my biopsy until I went to a second surgeon for a second opinion on my surgeon's pretty drastic recommendation.

"What if we just watch this?" I asked. (It was one of the options I'd discussed with my oncologist.)

I wrote down the second surgeon's answer: "Left alone this will kill you." I thought about the words often when I considered my own options, including the easy way out! His words came back, and they made a difference -- I didn't go the easy route.

Don't forget to bring copies of your pathology and DNA reports -- and even your mammogram if appropriate -- to your second opinion appointments.

THE NATIONAL CANCER INSTITUTE

Call the National Cancer Institute (1-800-4-CANCER) and ask its Cancer Information Service for the latest about your type of breast cancer. NCI has developed a Physician Data Query (PDQ) which also gives up-to-date treatment information to doctors. When you call NCI's number, you'll talk to a technician who will send you information on anything new happening with your type of cancer.

Also request any of the NCI's very good, and free, booklets that might pertain to you. These include:

Breast Cancer: Understanding Treatment Options
Radiation Therapy: A Treatment for Early Stage Breast Cancer
Mastectomy: A Treatment for Breast Cancer
Breast Reconstruction: A Matter of Choice
What You Need to Know about Breast Cancer.

NCI doesn't fool around getting this information to you. The materials you order will be in your mail in no time.

NCI has other booklets available, including ones to help your family cope with this crisis, to tell you about life after breast cancer, and even a somewhat scary booklet, *Chemotherapy and You*. Since this booklet covers chemo treatments for all types and stages of cancer, it's pretty heavy reading. Find out what course of chemo treatment your doctor advises before reading this booklet, because many of the problems cited in it will not occur during the typical courses of adjuvant chemotherapy given for early breast cancer.

Anyway, let this wonderful organization help you!

RELATIVES, FRIENDS, ORGANIZATIONS AND STRANGERS

If you have a relative who is a doctor, call him or her for advice and other resources for second opinions on your course of treatment. Get in touch with any relatives or friends you know who have had breast cancer for their ideas and opinions. If you don't know anybody who has actually experienced breast cancer, ask your doctor, your doctor's nurse, and relatives and friends for the names of people who have had cancer similar to yours.

Don't be afraid to call anybody who is recommended. By its very nature, breast cancer produces a sisterhood among women who are survivors of the disease, and most of them will be more than happy to talk to you.

Besides local hospitals and clinics, there are many other organizations offering help. Such groups may assist, for instance, by providing the names and numbers of women who are willing to discuss their own experiences. Among these associations is the Y-ME National Organization for Breast Cancer Information and Support which produces, among other things, an outstanding newsletter with the latest in breast cancer news. Call 1-800-221-2141 or look under "My Image" (after Breast Cancer), Y-ME's affiliate local organization, in your phone book. My Image offers local meetings and support systems, as well as the names of cancer patients willing to discuss their experiences with breast cancer.

The National Breast Cancer Coalition, founded by noted breast surgeon and author Susan Love, is an activist group aimed at establishing funding and priorities for breast cancer research. You can write the Coalition at 1707 L Street, N.W., Washington, D.C. 20036, or call 202-296-7477.

Another source of information and support is the National Alliance of Breast Cancer Organizations (NABCO), telephone 212-719-0154.

If you are thinking about reconstruction, especially immediate reconstruction, ask your plastic surgeon to give you the names of some previous patients so that you can find out how these women feel about the results of their procedures. The same goes for radiation and chemotherapy. You won't be given the names of anybody who's going to hang up on you; you'll only be referred to women who are willing to talk about their own experiences.

LIBRARIES AND BOOKSTORES

Browse through bookstores and libraries to see if there are any books or periodicals that might be of special interest to you. If you don't mind somewhat technical reading, ask your librarian for the indexes of recent copies of *The New England Journal of Medicine*, the *Journal of the American Medical Association (JAMA)*, *Journal of the National Cancer Institute*, or *The Lancet*, a respected British publication, and you can look up articles relating to breast cancer. *The Merck Manual of Diagnosis and Therapy*, published by Merck Research Laboratories, is now the most widely used medical text in the world![82]

Some easier reading might include *Choices: Realistic Alternatives in Cancer Treatment* by Marion Morra & Eve Potts, Avon Books, 1987, an excellent book giving an overview of cancer.

Dr. Susan Love's Breast Book with Karen Lindsey, Addison-Wesley Publishing Co., Inc., 1990 & 1991, (revised 1995) is one of the best around. Dr. Love gives a thorough and compassionate look at various treatments for breast cancer, with interesting comments on alternative medicine, treatment of cancers in situ, and the role of diet and cancer. She also has some controversial comments on the value of breast self-exams. (I disagree with her here!)

Another good book is *Breast Cancer/The Complete Guide* by Yashar Hirshaut, M.D. F.A.C.P., and Peter I. Pressman, M.D. F.A.C.S., Bantam Books, 1992. Among other positives, these doctors offer considerable hope for patients with breast cancer recurrence.

If you like your reading on the lighter side, try *My Breast*, by Joyce Wadler, Addison-Wesley Publishing Co., 1992, the humorous and interesting account of one woman's battle with early breast cancer. Ms. Wadler makes CMF chemotherapy sound like a breeze, but she did her research and the reader will learn as well as laugh.

There are many other books available, including the "classics" by Betty Rollin and Rose Kushner which helped change attitudes towards breast cancer treatment.

Some books with a more emotional or basic angle include *Spinning Straw Into Gold/Your Emotional Recovery from Breast Cancer*, by Ronnie Kaye (an L.A. psychotherapist), Lamppost Press, Simon & Schuster, 1991; *The Breast Cancer Companion* by Kathy LaTour (anecdotal in tone with lots of "tips"), William Morrow & Co., 1993; *The Breast Cancer Handbook/Taking Control After You've Found a Lump* by Joan Swirsky & Barbara Balaban (some basics), HarperPerennial, 1994.

THE MOMENT OF TRUTH

The time will come when you have to make a decision about your treatment options. You've done your research, you've asked questions of your doctors and nurses, you've talked to other women who have faced breast cancer. Your doctors, and those close to you, can help you with the choices you must make, but the final decision is up to you. You are your Most Important Advocate. Go for it!

13. COPING

Let's face facts -- it ain't easy. Almost half of breast cancer patients develop some sort of "adjustment disorder," according to Carol L. Alter, director of psychosocial services at the Temple University Comprehensive Cancer Center in Philadelphia. And twenty percent of these patients have even more serious disturbances, primarily depression, Dr. Alter reported.[83]

It's natural to feel a sense of disbelief and denial when you are diagnosed with breast cancer. Then along come depression and anxiety. Finally -- in about two to four weeks after the diagnosis, according to Dr. Alter -- a "normal" patient adjusts to her situation.

But the ordeal has just begun. "All people who have been diagnosed with cancer have high probabilities of experiencing anger, fear, and anxiety," says Katherine A. Billingham, PhD, writing in the *Y-ME Hotline Newsletter*.[84]

According to *The London Sunday Times Magazine,* "Something like 25% of [British] breast patients go into clinical depression following breast surgery."[85] And then, for many of us, there is chemotherapy to boot! You owe it to yourself to put together mechanisms that will help you to cope.

It's also normal for any woman to continue to be anxious even after surgery, and there doesn't seem to be much difference in the anxiety factor between women having a lumpectomy and those having a mastectomy. After all, we are all facing a dangerous enemy! The question we need to answer is how to get on with our lives.

DEALING WITH YOUR FEELINGS

1. PUTTING TOGETHER YOUR SUPPORT GROUP

You are going to need people to talk to about this crisis in your life. Some women prefer one-on-one relationships; others like the dynamics available in a support group. It doesn't matter what kind of support you have; just remember you really do need someone to talk to about the problems you are facing and your day-to-day experiences with your surgery, radiation, and chemo. You also need some people who have experienced, or are experiencing, these problems themselves.

The first thing I did after I flunked my biopsy was to call Eileen Guzikowski. I'd known her for many years but we had never been really close friends. I knew, however, that she had had breast cancer and we had talked about her trials with chemotherapy. Eileen was great. When I asked if she had any emotion that stood out from the others, she replied, "Stark terror."

Her words were the right ones to hear because what had been my primary emotion? The same: stark terror.

Eileen was wonderful, candid and caring. She told me that all those feelings I was experiencing -- anger, fear, grief -- were normal. Our deepening friendship was one of the best things to come out of my own experience with breast cancer. I was also glad that my friend Amy, whom you'll read about later, had shared her battles with me.

While trying to find some women who had had my particular type of adjuvant chemotherapy, I became friends with Barbara Gillies, another patient of my own doctor, who gave me good tips about coping with chemo. And, thanks to the experience of a friend of a friend, I decided to have immediate reconstruction. Plus, sharing breast cancer concerns renewed a close friendship with my college classmate Phyllis Beardsley.

It was also comforting to know that some of my family members had put me on their "prayer list." The rector of

Grace Episcopal Church in Kilmarnock, Va., says it is important to pray for others -- and comforting to those "others" if you let them know what and how you are doing.

Your own support "group" can be composed of one-on-one individuals or you can join one or more support groups in your area. These groups meet most often at clinics or hospitals. Your doctor or nurse should be able to give you the names of some such groups. You'll find others listed in this chapter.

Some experts feel strongly that every woman diagnosed with breast cancer should talk to a psychiatrist at some time during treatment. This is certainly an option if support groups don't fill the bill for you.

The American Cancer Society or the "Look Good...Feel Better" Program will have information about coping with emotional and physical problems. The American Cancer Society's local number will be in your phone book. Contact "Look Good...Feel Better" at 1-800-395-LOOK.

It may be particularly important for you to talk one-on-one with women who have had the kind of treatment you plan to undergo. The American Cancer Society's Reach to Recovery Program can put you in touch with such women, and, of course, you should feel free to ask your doctor or nurse for the names and numbers of patients who have undergone treatment similar to the one recommended for you.

Relatives or friends who have dealt with cancer may also help you. Cancer has come out of the closet. The worst thing you can do to yourself is to try to find one to hide in. Don't put your head in the sand. You are not an ostrich; you are a woman who needs all the support and love she can get. Don't try to "tough it out" alone.

You may also find, however, that your relationship with your husband or lover has never been closer. I think many of us are surprised at how little a breast plays in a husband's feelings for us. Basically, they want us to *live*! But this is a very stressful time for your immediate family. There is the anxiety, the trauma of your treatment, and, possibly, both psychological and physical effects on your sex life. Discuss such problems as vaginal dryness with your gynecologist. Remember that the trauma of your disease can intensify any existing problems in relationships. Your children and even your husband may be not only fearful but angry -- at you!

You may want to involve your husband or significant other and even your children in some sort of therapy program.

2. DEALING WITH DEPRESSION

Use your support people or group to help you through these tough times. If you need additional help, see a shrink -- or a member of the clergy. Talk to your doctor about your feelings and ask about people who may be able to help you. All your feelings are normal. This is a big deal emotionally, and nobody expects you to be perfect. If anybody does insist on perfection, he or she may not belong in your life at this time.

"Twenty years ago, the prognosis for cancer patients was so grim that the few therapists who worked with them focused solely on death and dying," Elisabeth Rosenthal wrote in *The New York Times* after an interview with psychiatrist Jimmie Holland. As an example of this attitude, Dr. Holland told *The Times*:

"The patient would say, 'Doctor, I've lost all my ability to have sex,' and the doctor would say, 'You're lucky to be alive.'"[86]

Now, thank God, that attitude is changing, and more doctors are treating the whole patient, not just the cancer.

If you are having trouble sleeping, ask for a mild anti-anxiety drug such as Ativan, which has relatively few side effects. Your doctor may prescribe something stronger if you need it, although some physicians seem to approach the cancer treatment process as an Outward Bound Program. It is sometimes mind-boggling to find that the same physician who is willing to subject you to the Big Three cancer treatments (cutting, burning and poisoning) is scared stiff to give you a pain pill or something that will help you sleep! If your doctor seems determined to ignore the emotional side of your treatment, try to get another physician or at least see a therapist. If you are in a health program where your options are limited, try to switch to another doctor within the group for your primary care.

Occasionally, you may find yourself very angry at your doctor over nothing. This, too, is pretty normal. Have you heard the expression, "Depression is anger turned inward?" In this case your anger is at the person or persons who appear to be making you miserable while taking your money. These feelings should pass, and your doctor should have the good sense to take your behavior in stride.

Your spouse or significant other may also experience depression or anger at the situation, or, sometimes, at the loss of your hair or your breast. If the two of you can't work things out, you may need outside help. Your children may also experience depression and acute anxiety. And who can blame them?

Give yourself some "fun" objectives. If you are having surgery, have something exciting to do after when you've recuperated. If you are having chemotherapy, plan your "rest periods" so you'll have something to look forward to. With radiation, plan a celebration when treatment is finished.

DEALING WITH YOUR BODY IMAGE

MASTECTOMY

For many women, the loss of a breast is as traumatic as the idea of breast cancer itself. This cruel loss can even obscure the "real" issue: the life-threatening nature of breast cancer itself.

There is the trauma of sharing your "new look" with your husband or lover. Take heart. When "Dear Abby" printed a column about one woman's despondency over her breast loss, the response from readers was surprisingly positive: Women of all ages wrote, in essence, that mastectomy was by no means the end of the world. As one reader put it, "A real man is interested in the person the woman is. If all he wants is a pair of 'boobs,' what kind of woman would be interested in him?"[87]

Bad as mastectomy may seem even today, things were worse when the radical Halsted was standard treatment. Nowadays there is usually much less scarring, and prosthesis and appropriate bras are much more sophisticated. The Reach to Recovery program and My Image (part of the Y-Me organization) are among the resources available for information and even, in some cases, prosthesis and bras. You can also ask your doctor or nurse for the names of stores specializing in supplies for mastectomy patients.

In their book, *Choices: Realistic Alternatives in Cancer Treatment*, Marion Morra and Eve Potts urge women not to shop alone for a prosthesis. They suggest you take an "involved person, such as your sister, mother, husband, or a good friend" along. They also suggest that you try on a variety of breast forms in order to determine what really is best for you.[88]

(See additional comments in Surgery chapter.)

Another breast "image" problem is radiation, which may leave the breast red and even cause blisters. Any areas exposed to radiation need extra lotions and should be kept out of the sun. Use sunscreen as well as lotions (especially those with aloe and Vitamin E).

HAIR LOSS

Hair loss is just about the hardest thing to take in chemotherapy. Losing one's hair may be the first time some breast cancer patients, especially those who did not experience breast loss, really confront their disease. Most chemotherapy

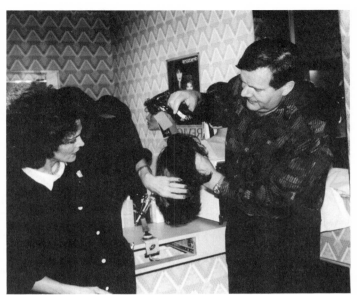

*Eivind Bjerke and Gloria Sansone prepare a wig
for a cancer patient as part of their work for
the "Look Good...Feel Better" program.*

programs will cause at least a thinning of the hair, and only a miracle will save total hair loss if you are given much Adriamycin. If you are going to have total hair loss, it usually comes early on in the treatment. And, if it does occur, you can wear a wig more comfortably than with hair remaining underneath.

Because hair is so important to most women -- and because its loss is such an outward sign of an inward misery -- it is essential to find ways to cope with the problem.

Philip Kingsley, a respected hair consultant, put it this way in *Vogue* Magazine: "...if your hair's not looking the way you want it to look, you actually don't feel good. It's deeply psychological. I've had women and men who are almost suicidal because they're losing their hair or it's not the way they want it to be. And that's not as unusual as one may think."[88]

After all, people even say, "I'm having a bad hair day."

Synthetic wigs are easier to take care of, are usually cheaper, and can look very natural. Get your hair cut very short while it is falling out. If possible, see a hairdresser who knows about the effects of chemotherapy. Turbans or scarves, some with clever "bangs" you can clip in, are helpful for times when you don't want to wear a wig.

Hair loss, unfortunately, is not confined to the head. You may also lose some or all of your eyelashes and eyebrows, pubic hair, etc. Programs like "Look Good...Feel Better" (see below) can help you learn to "feather" eyebrows on with an eye crayon and use a mascara wand on thinning eyelashes.

Remember, hard as it is, that hair loss is *temporary*. Your hair will return, sometimes thicker and more attractive than it ever was. Many people report their straight hair coming back curly. Others say the hair comes in darker, and if it had started going gray, may return in its original color.

ORGANIZATIONAL HELP

Ask about the "Look Good...Feel Better" program, developed by the Cosmetic, Toiletry, and Fragrance Association Foundation, the National Cosmetology Association, and the American Cancer Society. Call 1-800-395-LOOK or your local American Cancer Society for more information. Other programs that can help you cope include Y-ME, the National Organization for Breast Cancer Information and Support, headquartered in Chicago. Call 1-800-221-2141 or look in your local phone book for information. My Image (After Breast Cancer) is an affiliate organization offering local meetings and support systems.

If you should experience problems with lymphedema (swelling of the arm after lymph node surgery), you can get information from the National Lymphedema Network, 2211 Post Street, Suite 404, San Francisco CA 94115. Or call 1-800-541-3259.

"Meals on Wheels" may provide your solution to food shopping and cooking while you are recuperating. Most cities also have visiting nurse programs. Your hospital's social services unit may help you find nursing care.

Whatever problems you face, remember that you are far from alone! There are at least 1.5 million women with breast cancer in this country, and the majority of them are going to survive this earthquake in their lives. So try to get on with your life. Join that support group! Use that foundation! See that shrink! Talk to your minister or rabbi! And remember, knowledge is power. Know your illness. Keep going as much as possible. Don't be afraid to cry, and be willing to smile! It can't hurt.

Look to this day,
For it is life,
The very life of life.
In its brief course lie all
The realities and verities
    of existence,
The bliss of growth,
The splendor of action,
The glory of power.

For yesterday is but a dream,
And tomorrow is only a vision.
But today, well lived,
Makes every yesterday a dream
    of happiness
And every tomorrow a vision
    of hope.

Look well, therefore, to this day.

Sanskrit Proverb

From <u>Taking Time</u>,
National Cancer Institute

14. WHEN TREATMENT ENDS

Although reaching the end of treatment, especially if you have adjuvant radiation or chemotherapy, can seem as though it will never come, it does. Now comes the moment to get out the champagne and, after the celebration, to get on with your life.

Of course, you won't be fading into the woodwork: Your doctor will want to see you at least once every three months or so for the first two or three years. At these exams he or she will examine your breasts, your scars, the lymph nodes around your neck, collarbone and underarms, and will order blood work. These blood tests may include a CBC (complete blood count) that measures your white and red blood cells, another one that checks your kidney and liver functions, and possibly a CEA (carcinoembryonic antigen), a test which measures an antigen that frequently increases when breast cancer tumors are present. (An antigen is any foreign body that triggers a response in the immune system.)

If you had a lumpectomy or segmental mastectomy with radiation, you'll probably have a mammogram every six months for at least a couple of years. Once a year you will probably receive more extensive tests, including a mammogram, chest x-ray, urinalysis, and often an EKG (heart function test). Some doctors recommend an occasional bone scan or at least a baseline one at the time of your diagnosis.

The problem with bone scans is that they are not always perfect and may be unnecessarily alarming. As recently as 1991, the *Journal of the American Medical Association* noted that, "...only one in nine patients who have abnormal bone scans will be found to have bone metastases...The use of bone scan surveillance to detect recurrence has not been fruitful in asymptomatic patients."[90] You can imagine the anxiety such abnormal scans produced in the nine out of ten patients who were "normal."

Bone scans are not always accurate even when cancer has spread. A friend of mine who was experiencing pain in some of her ribs had a bone scan. Imagine her shock and terror when, after reading the scan, her doctor announced, "The cancer has spread all over your bones!" It turned out the cancer had indeed spread, but only to one area of her ribs. Even after $7,000 worth of tests, radiologists disagreed about a suspicious spot on her spine. (My friend is now in remission after more chemotherapy.)

Medical opinion is building that perhaps intensive follow-up is unnecessary unless a patient experiences symptoms. Two recent Italian clinical trials showed that frequent lab tests, x-rays, and bone scans did not improve survival rates or quality of life. One of the studies, in Florence, Italy, showed that intensive follow-up including chest x-rays and photos, and bone scans every six months, made no difference in five-year survival rates. The authors of this study recommended that chest x-rays and bone scans should be "limited to patients with suspicious symptoms or findings at periodic clinical examination, which should be recommended as the optimal follow-up procedure."[91]

Depending on your age and medical history, your physician may also order other tests at your annual physical, perhaps including an occult blood test and/or sigmoidoscopy, which check for colon cancer, and/or a pelvic vaginal ultrasound exam that can catch ovarian cancers and cysts. (Women with breast cancer history have a higher risk of both these diseases.)

Women taking tamoxifen as adjuvant therapy should see their gynecologist twice a year because of the increased risk of uterine cancer, as well as the possibility of other problems such as ovarian cysts and a thickening of the wall of the uterus.

Since 60% of breast cancer recurrences happen in the first three years after diagnosis, you will probably see your doctor on a three month, or, at most, a six-month schedule until your three years are up. Ironically, that's about the length of time it takes to get over the terror associated with these examinations!

A FEW PSYCHOLOGICAL NEGATIVES
After Treatment Depression
The most surprising thing about finishing your treatment may be how you feel once it is over. The National Cancer Institute notes this in its booklet, *After Breast Cancer*: "During treatment you had frequent, perhaps daily contact with your health care team. Many women say that when their treatment ends, they feel they have lost the support of some of those who were most involved with their physical needs....Until now, coping with treatment may have consumed much of your physical and mental energy. Yet, many women find that the demands of treatment were somehow reassuring. At least they were doing something to fight the cancer."

My friend Eileen Guzikowski had warned me about the possibility of feeling depressed once treatment was over, but that seemed pretty far out to me. "Just get me out of chemo and I'll be ready to take on the world," I thought.

My last chemotherapy treatment was in mid-October; my last blood test connected with chemo was at the end of the "rest period" two weeks later. To my surprise, instead of facing the upcoming holidays with enthusiasm, I was engulfed in gloom. Would this Thanksgiving, this Christmas, be my last?

I began to think more about cancer than I ever had while I was undergoing all the treatments. Every pain meant a return of the disease. While I had managed to lead an almost normal life during my chemotherapy, I now found coping more difficult.

Eventually I learned that this was a common reaction to the end of treatment. Much as you hate the surgery, the radiation and/or the chemotherapy, you know that it is helping you. Your condition is constantly monitored; you are a "regular" at the clinic, hospital, doctor's office. You may be on a first name basis with the lab technicians who draw your blood, the radiation therapists, the nurses and even the doctors who administer your treatments. No cancer cell would *dare* pop up with all those people looking after you!

Then it all ends. Suddenly you are on your own. Oh, you might be taking tamoxifen, but that's only a pill. The very complaints that you had about surgery, radiation or chemotherapy are at the heart of your new feelings. At least the discomfort and/or disfigurement meant that something was being *done* about your illness. Now people are no longer hovering over you, assisting you through each day.

I found that support groups didn't help at this time, either. There I was, surrounded by people with cancer. Of course, my feelings weren't helped by the deaths of four close friends and relatives, from various diseases, during this time. I wanted to get away from it all.

And a trip turned out to be "just what the doctor ordered" for me. My husband and I vacationed in the Provence section of France, and for the first time in over a year I forgot about cancer. Sometimes a vacation at the end of the treatment process is a good idea. You've been unable to get very far from home during your treatment, so it's time. Like my friend Eileen, I've found a new joy in traveling.

After-treatment depression will pass, but it is so common that you should be aware that it might happen. Some women feel that this is the time to see a therapist.

Sometimes sex can be a problem during and after chemotherapy in particular. If sex doesn't seem to be what it was before your treatments, tell your gynecologist. Try vaginal lubricants a couple of times a week. You might also get your testosterone tested. Yes, that's a male hormone but we have it, too. You might even need a supplement of it!

But Was It a Cure?

Unless your cancer was diagnosed as particularly aggressive, the chances are you were so wrapped up in the terror and torments of the moment, biopsies, surgery, radiation, chemotherapy, that the ultimate possible result of all this -- death -- seemed far away. Then you are finished with your treatments. Everything has been done that can be done. So now what? This may be the first time that you consider that future possibilities could include your own mortality. Such thoughts can be pretty immobilizing.

One way to deal with this is to do something positive about these negative feelings. Perhaps this is a good time to get your spiritual life in order. And take the time to let the people you love know how much you love them.

On a more practical level, do you have a will? If not, get one. Do you have a living will, a document that indicates you do not want life-support systems or other extraordinary life-saving procedures if you become too ill to make such decisions for yourself? On a particularly dismal day you might plan what funeral arrangements you want, if you want any. Write a brief biography about yourself. Determine your net worth.

It never hurts to have these projects done, even if you live to be a hundred. And why not get them out of the way while you are healthy? (Albeit depressed.)

If these ideas don't turn you on, pretend that you only have one year of healthy living left and make a list of things you would most like to do if that was all the time you had left. Then DO some of them now!

Remember, too, that exercise is one of the best ways to get depressing thoughts out of your mind. Jog. Do aerobics. Clean out your closets. And remember that the odds are you *are* going to beat the disease.

TERROR AT EXAM TIMES

Be prepared to feel anxious whenever an exam is coming up. This is perfectly natural. Between 80 to 90 percent of cancer patients experience fear, anxiety and anger for up to two or more years after their diagnosis.

The physician you see may depend in part on the type of treatment you have; for example, you may return to your radiologist if you had adjuvant radiation therapy, or to your oncologist if you had chemotherapy. Most surgeons also want to perform occasional exams after your operation(s).

If you have a symptom that you think might be cancer-related, don't hesitate to call your doctor, especially if it lasts more than a couple of weeks. Pain is one symptom that worries breast cancer survivors, especially since it could indicate cancer in the bones. Remember, however, that when breast cancer spreads, it generally goes to the ribs or to big bones such as the hips, pelvis, backbone or the upper parts of the extremities. This means that your painful ankle or wrist and your aching elbow are usually ineligible for the worry list. Chances are, too, that your lower back pain is something you'd get anyway, but if it lasts more than a couple of weeks, check it out. Remember that most people have back problems at some time in their lives. And many of us have arthritis as well.

Stomach pain doesn't necessarily mean your liver is on the blink, and you will have regular blood tests and a physical exam to check on it anyway.

A headache doesn't mean you have a brain tumor, but if you have a persistent dull ache that lasts more than a couple of weeks, or if you start experiencing double vision, then have it checked out. (Of course, that nagging headache may also be a sinus infection.)

Don't worry about the cough that comes along with a bad cold or flu. But remember, if you're feeling really sick or have a fever, you should see a doctor anyway, particularly if your cough is producing yellow or green sputum. This could indicate the kind of infection that can turn into bronchitis or pneumonia. A dry non-productive cough that lingers more than two weeks should be checked out.

Doctors generally count "recurrence-free" time from the date your cancer was treated by the surgery which removed it. Some doctors count cancer-free time from the end of any later adjuvant treatment such as radiation or chemotherapy.

AND NOW THE POSITIVE...

Consider today to be the first day of your new, post-treatment life. Use the positives in your life -- people, prayer, productivity, play -- to fulfill your joy in it. Get on with living!

15. WHAT ABOUT
RECURRENCE?

We are all haunted by the fear of recurrence. What we have to remember is that fear is deadly. As psychiatrist Julia Rowland and social worker Deborah Dozier-Hall put it to a group of cancer survivors, fear can wipe out your life before cancer ever does.[92]

THE ODDS

Although breast cancer cells can have a history of popping up in another tumor years after the original diagnosis, the odds are that the longer you go without a recurrence the greater your chances are of not having one. Sixty percent of recurrences are within the first three years of diagnosis and 20 percent are within the next two years.

The statistics for both recurrence and mortality are confusing and lag behind what is actually happening. But now, for the first time in decades, "There has been a clear decline in deaths due to breast cancer in American women," Samuel Broder, retiring head of the National Cancer Institute, announced in January 1995. From 1989 to 1992 the death rate for white women has declined 6 percent.

"From 1987 to 1992 there has been a roughly 18 percent decline in the death rate for white women aged 30 to 39," Dr. Broder said. Other decreases in white women were:

Ages 40 to 49 -- 8.1 percent decrease
Ages 50 to 59 -- 9.3 percent decrease
Ages 60 to 69 -- 4.8 percent decrease
Ages 70 to 79 -- 3.4 percent decrease.

Unfortunately, African-American women have not experienced this decline. "Thus, breast cancer is another example of a disease against which there is a differential course of progress in our society," Dr. Broder added.[93]

Similar concerns about cancer and Afro-Americans came up at a conference of the American Public Health Association. "The impact of cancer on black Americans constitutes a major public health crisis," according to Ruth McCorkle, PhD.

At the same meeting, Beverly Rhine, with the Women of Color Breast Cancer Survivors Support Project in Compton, CA, urged the use of African-American churches as a site for breast cancer education and screening.[94]

Here are a few breast cancer statistics:

The five-year survival for Stage I breast cancer in all women is over 90 percent.

Fifty-three percent of all white breast cancer patients are diagnosed as Stage I. This group has at least an 80 percent five-year survival rate, while only 42 percent of all black breast cancer patients are diagnosed with Stage I cancer and only 62 percent of them reach the five-year mark, according to Dr. Devra Lee Davis, Science Advisor to the Public Health Service.

Breast cancer is basically a disease of older women; 80 percent of those diagnosed are over 50.

According to one study, the five-year survival rates for the various stages of cancer in all women of all ages are:

- Local (no spread to nodes) 92.7%
- Regional (spread to nodes) 71.1%
- Distant (spread to other
  parts of the body)   17.8%
- Stage unknown   50.15%

Remember that statistics lag far behind facts. It takes from seven to 15 years for numbers to reflect the results of incidence, diagnosis, treatments. Today's facts may be considerably better than yesterday's figures.

Fortunately, the symptoms of something that could indicate a recurrence or metastasis are usually indicative of something else -- a head cold, the flu, menopause, arthritis. Nonetheless, according to the National Cancer Institute, you should watch out for certain symptoms and discuss them with your doctor, especially if they continue for more than a week or so:

● Changes in your breast or the scar area, including lumps, redness, swelling, and tiny hard pimple-like nodules

● Pain in your breast, shoulder, hips, lower back or the pelvic area

● Coughing or hoarseness

● Nausea, vomiting, diarrhea or heartburn lasting more than a few days

● Loss of appetite or unexplained weight changes

● Changes in your menstrual cycle or flow

● Dizziness, blurred vision, severe or frequent headaches, problems with walking.

LOCAL RECURRENCE
"No one dies from local recurrence," Dr. Colleen Hagen writes.[95]

A local recurrence means that the cancer has returned to the area where it first happened, such as, in the case of lumpectomy, in the breast itself. Or it may turn up in the lymph nodes under the arm. Five to 30 percent of women with radical or modified radical mastectomies will also experience a recurrence in the area of the surgery. Some doctors feel that since all the breast tissue was taken out, this cancer is very serious because it had to find its way back through the blood or lymph node system to make a reappearance. However, the *Journal of the National Cancer Institute*[96] reported on an Italian study that indicated some tumor cells that get left behind can lie dormant in the area for years and then begin to grow rapidly.

The recurring cancer in the breast region may take the form of one or more nodules, or small pimples. These can be treated by radiation to the area, particularly if the woman has had a mastectomy. If a tumor or nodules occur in the breast after a lumpectomy and radiation, the patient may have to have a mastectomy. (You can only give so much radiation to one area of the body because your tissues can only stand so much "burn.")

Even if the new cancer is found in the other breast, it is regarded more as a new or "second primary tumor" rather than as a "distant metastatic" one. If you should develop cancer of the other breast, your treatment will be similar to what you would have undergone if this had been your first experience with breast cancer. If you have a regional recurrence or cancer in the other breast, you'll go "back to the drawing board" and have the same tests you had originally to determine the stage of the cancer, and to make sure it has not spread. Once the tests are done and evaluated, you will treatment -- probably surgery, radiation, and/or chemotherapy -- based on the results.

DISTANT METASTATIC DISEASE

If cancer spreads beyond the breast and surrounding lymph nodes, it is called a distant metastasis. Without adjuvant chemotherapy and/or tamoxifen, some women with Stage II breast cancer could have a 40 to 80 percent chance of developing metastatic disease.

The most common sites for cancer spread are the scalp, the lungs, liver, bones, and brain. Since breast cancer is a systemic disease; that is, it spreads through the lymph and blood systems, the chances are that once a cancer shows up at a distant site, it may have spread to other places as well. Before beginning treatment, doctors usually do a battery of tests to try to determine if there is any other site involved.

TREATMENT OPTIONS

Sometimes, if the metastasis is found in only one spot, the cancer may be cured by removing it or zapping it with radiation. Although many doctors feel that metastatic breast cancer is not curable, they do believe that it can be put into remission; i.e., the cancer symptoms disappear, sometimes for many years. In other cases treatment may be palliative; that is, it may relieve or lesson the symptoms.

THE POSSIBILITY OF CURE

Some medical professionals are more optimistic about cure. "The best approach to treating a recurrence of breast cancer is to devise a strategy that...puts the first and primary emphasis, wherever possible, on trying for cure," write Doctors Yashar Hirshaut and Peter I. Pressman.[97]

If the interval between the original cancer and the new metastasis is more than two years and the original tumor was fairly small, patients are often treated with another dose of their original chemotherapy, or they may be given a stronger set of chemo goodies. A patient who had been given CMF (cyclophosphamide, methotrexate and 5-fluorouracil) may be switched to a more potent chemo combination such as CAF, where doxorubicin (Adriamycin) is substituted for methotrexate. A clinical trial is now studying CAF versus CAF plus leucovorin. (See Chemotherapy chapter for more information on these drugs.) Many doctors give a combination of chemo and hormone therapy. Some more rigorous chemo drugs used in recurring cancer are Thiotepa, Cisplatin, vinblastine, Mitoxanthrone, Mitomycin-C, and VP-16.

In a study comparing the potent CAF with less rigorous chemotherapy, researchers at the Comprehensive Cancer Center at Wake Forest University, N.C., found no difference in survival rates nor did shorter periods of chemotherapy result in poorer survival in women with metastatic breast cancer. Two women on the CAF protocol died of sepsis (infection) according to the study, published in *The New England Journal of Medicine*.[98] Nonetheless, if you develop distant metastatic breast cancer, you will probably receive a more rigorous chemotherapy.

Even women 70 and over can benefit from chemotherapy for metastatic breast cancer in terms of response, survival and toxic effects, according to a study by the Piedmont Oncology Association, reported in the *Journal of the American Medical Association*.[99]

HORMONAL DRUGS

Women who are hormone-receptive may receive endocrine therapy, or drugs that involve the hormonal system, such as tamoxifen or aminoglutethimide. Doctors have a number of these drugs to use; the drugs are usually given in sequence -- when one drug stops working, the next one is tried.

Tamoxifen is the preferred first drug and can be effective in halting metastatic cancer for a year or more. On the other hand, patients already taking tamoxifen as adjuvant therapy will be taken off the drug, since it's obviously no longer doing its job. When tamoxifen loses its power, doctors may prescribe aminoglutethimide (Cytadren), which works through the adrenal gland, reducing the estrogen-like properties that gland produces. Cytadren, however, lowers the adrenal gland's manufacture of cortisone, so patients taking the drug are also usually given steroids to make up for the loss of cortisone.

Next in line is Halotestin (fluoxymesterone), an "androgenic," or male hormone, which seems effective in treating cancer of the bone, although it can cause the development of male characteristics (such as excess facial hair) and may cause an excess of calcium in the blood.

Megace (megestrol) is effective in women who have progesterone positive receptors. Megace may cause weight gain and fluid retention.

Lupron (leuprolide acetate), also used in the treatment of prostate cancer, inhibits the pituitary gland, which also produces estrogen. Sometimes this drug will cause a "flare" of the original symptoms before it starts being effective.

RADIATION

Sometimes it is possible to use radiation alone to treat skin and/or bone cancers. Radiation therapy to the bone may provide not only relief from pain but strengthening of the bone as well, thus preventing spontaneous fractures.

EXPERIMENTAL DRUGS

More treatments are being developed all the time. And many women are willing to endure the side effects of experimental drugs in order to have even a slim chance of prolonging their lives. *The London Sunday Times Magazine* reported that the British Imperial Cancer Fund asked a group of healthy individuals as well as some medical professionals if they would be willing to tolerate the side effects of strong adjuvant chemotherapies. Only 19 percent of healthy people said they would agree to endure such side effects, as did only 20 percent of the oncologists, and 4.5 percent of radio-therapists. Yet, the article states, over half the cancer patients said "they would endure the most severe side-effects, even if there was only a 1% chance of cure."[100]

That's the beauty of the human condition. Hope *does* spring eternal.

In addition to the chemotherapies and hormonal drugs already described, additional treatments for metastatic breast cancer include the following:

BONE MARROW TRANSPLANTATION

This drastic treatment is usually only given when cancer has metastasized, but is sometimes also prescribed for Stage II patients with a poor prognosis, such as those with an aggressive cancer, significant lymph node involvement, or a strong family history of breast cancer.

In this procedure *really* high doses of chemotherapy are given to shrink any tumors. Sometimes bone marrow is donated, but a new procedure (autologous bone-marrow transplants or ABMT) uses the patient's own marrow. In this case the bone marrow is removed before the completion of treatment. (Many times doctors try to shrink the tumors significantly before attempting the transplant.) The marrow itself is treated to remove all traces of cancer, then frozen. The idea behind this is to preserve the health of the bone marrow, which manufactures all the elements of the blood (red cells, white cells, and platelets) destroyed by the use of high dose-intensive chemotherapy.

Meanwhile the patient receives chemotherapy and radiation to treat the cancer. When the patient has had enough chemotherapy and radiation necessary to remove all traces of cancer from her body, the marrow is thawed and injected into her system through an IV.

This treatment is drastic -- the patient is kept in isolation and protected from infection. You can't even wear a wig! Side effects can include severe liver and lung damage, and there is a 3 percent risk of death from the transplant alone.

Not everyone is enthusiastic about this experimental procedure.

Dennis P. Beck, the father of a young woman who died after a transplant for Hodgkin's disease, wrote *The Wall Street Journal* a bitter letter about "a procedure that turned my daughter's body into an Auschwitz clone, caused her to vomit blood and bile routinely, and did nothing for her cancer."[101]

On the other hand, I know at least two women who have survived these treatments beautifully. "My faith kept me going," says Dolores Waller. A woman in her forties, she also felt she had the will to endure because of her small daughter.

In a Duke University study, women surviving bone marrow transplants for a year reported few side effects and an adequate quality of life after treatment. Some did experience fatigue, but the most frequently mentioned side effect was a decrease in sexual interest and activity.[102]

Bone marrow transplants are risky, and they are extremely expensive, in some cases costing as much as $200,000! Many health insurers refuse to extend coverage for this procedure.

If you and your doctors feel that you could benefit from a bone marrow transplant, you should investigate the possibility of entering a clinical trial program. Such programs are available at various medical facilities as well as the National Institutes of Health. (See chapter on Clinical Trials.)

TAXOL

Taxol is a relatively new drug derived from the Pacific yew tree. In various trials it has shown remarkable ability to at least temporarily shrink the tumors of women with late-stage ovarian and breast cancers as well as to alleviate pain. It is now approved by the Food and Drug Administration for use in advanced ovarian cancer and for metastatic breast cancer patients who have experienced a relapse or were unresponsive to chemotherapy.

Although taxol has proved effective in about one fourth of ovarian cancer cases, its benefits may not last, and studies on how to make it more effective are underway. Although taxol lacks some of the severe side effects of such drugs as Adriamycin, it does cause hair loss, numbness, and sometimes temporary but intense pain occurring 2 to 4 days after treatment. A group of Italian scientists found that antihistamines can help control this pain.[103]

Research is underway to improve taxol itself and to find out if and how it works when used in conjunction with other chemotherapies. The National Cancer Institute has ongoing breast cancer trials to determine how much taxol to use and for how long.

Taxol has its detractors. "If this is the best new weapon in the war on cancer, maybe it's time to rethink our strategy," noted *Health* Magazine.[104]

NAVELBINE (VINORELBINE)

This drug, developed in France, produced a positive response in 163 of 354 women in six separate clinical trials in Europe and the United States, according to Charles L. Vogel, M.D., F.A.C.P., in the *Y-ME Hotline Newsletter*. It has fewer toxic effects than many other chemotherapy drugs and can also be used in combination with them.

"Because of its excellent response rates and subjective toxicity profile, single agent Navelbine could ultimately become the first line chemotherapeutic agent of choice for the palliative care of older women with metastatic disease and could become a valuable agent earlier in the course of breast cancer....," Dr. Vogel writes.[105]

Navelbine so far has not been granted approval by the FDA, in part because of its Oncology Drugs Advisory Committee's questions concerning cases of "significant worsening of cancer-related symptoms" and other problems.[106] Navelbine's manufacturer is conducting additional studies.

IMMUNE THERAPIES

One of the newest experiments in treating advanced breast cancer is to immunize patients against their own tumors. In other words, the immune system takes up the fight against the cancer. One of the ways to do this is to get the body's immune system to attack the kind of antigens, or markers, that show up in breast cancer cells. Usually the antibodies and white blood cells of the immune system attack antigens, but for some reason the antigens attached to breast cancer cells are often ignored by these fighters.

Studies of these and other vaccines are underway in the U.S., Canada, and Great Britain.

The Office of Alternative Medicine, part of the National Institutes of Health, is funding a study of 25 breast cancer patients to see if hypnosis and mental imagery can help boost the immune system.

METASTASES BLOCKER

The National Cancer Institute is currently running a clinical trial of carboxyamido-triazole to determine if the drug can stabilize tumor growth and block metastases. Preliminary results show the drug has few toxic side effects.

MAKING CANCER CELLS NORMAL

Scientists at McMaster University in Hamilton, Ontario, Canada, have identified an enzyme, telomerase, so far found only in cancer cells, which may help them become "immortal," allowing them to continue to grow while normal cells continue to live only a "normal" life span and die off. An inhibitor could cause cancer cells to lose their "immortality" and die like normal cells. Clinical trials to explore this are expected to start soon.[107]

ANTI-ANGIOGENIC AGENTS

Most tumors need a system of blood vessels (angiogenesis) to help them grow. Four anti-angiogenic agents, which could prevent the development of this blood vessel network, are now in clinical trials.[108]

ALTERNATIVE MEDICINE
Shark Cartilage Therapy?

Ask most oncoogists about shark cartilage therapy, and the most polite response you'd probably get would be a snort.

The idea behind shark cartilage is that it is supposed to inhibit the development of blood vessels that tumors need to grow and spread (angiogenesis). Dr. I. William Lane is not a cancer researcher, but his book, written with Linda Comac -- *Sharks Don't Get Cancer: How Shark Cartilage Could Save Your Life* -- is widely sold. The book claims that, in clinical trials in Mexico and Cuba, many terminally ill cancer patients experienced tumor reductions, and in some cases, remission of their tumors.

Medical News Director Mark Stern of the National Institutes of Health says that the therapy isn't proven and that the body doesn't absorb shark cartilage well enough to do any good. (A typical dosage is three capsules before each meal three times a day.)

But there was Art, who was diagnosed with metastatic kidney cancer in the spring of 1993. After powerful chemotherapy landed him in the hospital and it was obvious that he couldn't tolerate more such treatments, an oncologist gave him six weeks to live. Then Art heard from a friend with cancer, diagnosed as terminal the previous year, who was doing well on shark cartilage.

Art started taking the cartilage and lived another year and a half after the oncologist's prognosis. The large tumor on his rib cage shrank. Another oncologist, who treated him for the last year, told Art that his improvement probably *was* due to the shark cartilage he was taking.

This is anecdotal information only, since shark cartilage has not been proven effective in any controlled clinical trials within the American medical community. But many cancer patients do try treatments such as this, which are supported by books or well-meaning friends. Patients who undertake such alternative treatments should be sure to continue their regular medical care as well.

And, be advised that another friend, eventually cured of cancer after treatment at the National Institutes of Health, almost died from the vitamin overdose an "alternative therapist" had recommended.

PAIN

Pain control has become much more sophisticated in the last few years, but many patients still don't receive enough pain medicine, partly because both patients and doctors are unduly concerned about the addictiveness.

In a survey of over a thousand oncologists, more than 85 percent felt that most cancer patients were undermedicated for pain, according to Nessa Coyle, R.N., addressing a conference at the University of Minnesota. Between 40% and 80% of patients with advanced cancer don't receive enough pain relief, according to Ms. Coyle, director of the supportive care program of the department of neurology pain service at Memorial Sloan-Kettering Cancer Center.[109]

In addressing the medical profession's fear of drug addiction, Ms. Coyle pointed out that fewer than one percent of patients who receive narcotics for pain become psychologically dependent or addicted.

Another reason for controlling pain is that it can actually inhibit the body's immune system from doing its job.

"Unrelieved pain can produce unnecessary suffering, limit physical activity, decrease the appetite, reduce the amount of sleep, and increase the fear of cancer, all of which reduce the patient's ability to fight the disease," according to Ada Jacox, professor of nursing at The Johns Hopkins School of Nursing and co-chair of the Cancer Pain Guidelines Panel, speaking at a press conference on Management of Cancer Pain. The Cancer Pain Guideline Panel, sponsored by the federal Agency for Health Care Policy and Research, was convened to study cancer pain management and make recommendations on approaches to pain management.

Dr. Richard Payne, chief of the pain and symptom management section of the M.D. Anderson Cancer Center and co-chair of the Pain Panel, said that "...we have the necessary knowledge, if applied appropriately, to relieve even severe pain in most cancer patients."

He added that many patients are reluctant to talk about their pain "for fear of being labelled a 'complaining patient' and because they may not want to 'distract' the doctor from the equally important task of treating the cancer. Yet pain management is an essential part of overall cancer treatment." Dr. Payne also stressed that the use of opioid pain medications such as morphine is "the cornerstone of treatment of cancer pain, particularly when patients report severe pain. Physician *and* patient reluctance to prescribe and use medications such as morphine as early as necessary, and in the doses necessary to achieve pain control, are important contributors to the undertreatment of cancer pain."[110]

The guideline recommends a comprehensive approach to pain management, using surgery, radiation, nerve blocks and other treatments as needed for the best possible care.

You can obtain a copy of the *Cancer Pain Guideline* by calling 1-800-4-CANCER or writing Cancer Pain Guideline, P.O. Box 8547, Silver Spring, MD 20907.

Meantime, keep the following in mind:

● Almost all pain (90%) can be controlled.

● Many patients with advanced cancer may experience moderate to very severe pain. Plan for handling pain ahead of time.

● Admit pain to your doctor; he or she won't think you are "silly" or cowardly, but neither is your doctor a mind reader.

● Do not accept the myths that (1) you'll become addicted to your pain medication and (2) it will not work if you use it too often.

● What is NOT myth is that once pain is established, *more pain killer* is needed to control it.

● Not all cancer causes pain.

● Pain killers do not have to be given by injection.

• Like all drugs, pain killers can have side effects, including stomach upsets, constipation, sleepiness, nausea and dry mouth.

If you need medication for pain, speak up! Medications range from non-opioids such as Tylenol, Motrin and Advil, to opioids such as morphine, codeine, and hydromorphone for moderate to severe pain. Antidepressants and anticonvulsants can help control tingling and burning pain while steroids reduce pain caused by swelling.

Although most patients can be helped by oral pain medications, another development in managing pain is a pump (patient controlled analgesic device or PCA). This pump has a small needle which administers a regular dosage of medication intravenously. If the patient is in pain, she can boost her dose from time to time.

Specialists in nuclear medicine report advances in treatment of pain from tumors that have spread to the bone. Just as radiation to an affected area can help, so can drugs such as Phosphorus-32 or thophosphate (P-32), the first radio-pharmaceutical drug available in the USA for bone pain. Studies show an injection of another drug, Strontium-89, provides relief for as long as three months to 80 percent of patients. Strontium-99 is now under study by the Food and Drug Administration. These drugs appear to work by carrying radioactivity to the cancer site.

With so many drugs available there is no excuse for patients to suffer needless pain.

As oncologist Frederick P. Smith wrote in *The Washington Clinic Newsletter*, "...management of pain, with its consequent improvement in the quality of life, remains by far the primary challenge in maintaining longevity and the desire for living in our patients."[111]

16. CLINICAL TRIALS AND OTHER STUDIES

Although we often think of medical research as something occurring primarily in a laboratory, many of the treatments for, and statistics about, cancer and other diseases come from controlled studies and trials that use people, and these people are very often patients. Sometimes the study will be of a new drug or other treatment that is fresh from laboratory and/or animal testing, but other such studies may involve an "old" drug, food, or nutrient, testing to see if it can prevent (or cause) cancer or other ailments, or how it compares to a new or other treatment.

Clinical trials involving new drugs and other treatments are very precisely run programs established to show the effects of a treatment on a group of patients. These trials are divided into phases, and patients are eligible to participate in a given phase according to the extent and type of their illness, or in some cases, wellness.

The National Institutes of Health and cancer research centers throughout the country are among those using clinical trials to determine the value of standard and experimental treatments. Usually, the U.S. Food and Drug Administration only approves drugs such as new chemotherapies after they have been through a clinical trial.

Several groups throughout the country cooperate in various clinical trials for breast cancer research. Among the largest of these is the Nurses' Health Study, a research project sponsored by the Harvard School of Public Health and involving 200,000 nurses in various studies. Much of the information about cancer risk has evolved out of this project, started in 1976.

The Women's Health Initiative, launched by the National Institutes of Health, is the largest clinical trial of women ever conducted in the U.S. The randomized controlled part of the trial will include 63,000 women aged 50 to 79 from many ethnic and racial backgrounds and last for 15 years. The program will include controlled studies of what such factors as estrogen replacement therapy, low-fat diets, and vitamin supplements have on breast and colon cancer and heart disease.

THE NSABP TRIALS: TRIUMPHS AND TRIBULATIONS

Another large group is the National Surgical Adjuvant Breast & Bowel Project, which conducts clinical trials in breast and colorectal cancer research. NSABP, as it's called, was started in 1958, and is headquartered in Pittsburgh, Pa., and funded primarily by the National Cancer Institute with additional support from the American Cancer Society. The majority of NSABP members are located at non-university centers, allowing patients to participate in state-of-the-art clinical trials without having to travel great distances.

The NSABP trials were the first in America to show positively that mastectomy was no more effective than removal of part of the breast, that follow-up radiation lessened recurrence in the breast, that adjuvant chemotherapy could delay recurrence and increase survival rates, and that the hormonal drug tamoxifen also increased survival and delayed recurrence.

Then, in 1994, the *Chicago Tribune* published reports of flaws in the landmark mastectomy versus lumpectomy trial, published in 1985, the results of which had changed the course of breast cancer treatment in America. One of the principal researchers involved, a professor of surgery in Montreal, Canada, had falsified data, allowing 99 non-eligible women to participate in the study at Montreal's St. Luc Hospital. The doctor claimed that he allowed these women into the study for humanitarian reasons, and there is no evidence that he was trying to skew the results. But the 354 women from St. Luc Hospital did account for 16 percent of the total participants in this watershed trial.

Officials from the National Cancer Institute, the American Cancer Society, and the NSABP agreed that the St. Luc data could be eliminated and the end result would be the same. Nonetheless, news of the flawed study put a damper on it as well as three studies, one dealing with adjuvant chemotherapy and two with tamoxifen as adjuvant therapy with and without chemotherapy. St. Luc Hospital accounted for 14, 8, and 7 percent of the participants in these additional clinical trials.

Later, other discrepancies were found in the 1985 trial. And then, the NSABP study of tamoxifen (B-14), the positive preliminary results of which had been published in 1989, had its own problems. Evidence came to light that women taking tamoxifen in this study had eventually experienced an unusually high rate of endometrial cancer (cancer of the lining of the uterus). Four deaths had occurred from the disease, a highly unusual development with this cancer which is generally curable when caught early.

And that wasn't all. Women participating in another NSABP program, this one a study of tamoxifen as a preventative, had been given consent forms that stated no deaths from uterine cancer had been found in previous tamoxifen studies.

All these problems eventually led federal officials to undertake audits of the trials, disallow new participants in ongoing studies until the investigations were complete, and force the resignation of the distinguished head of the NSABP studies, Dr. Bernard Fisher. The National Institutes of Health, parent agency of the National Cancer Institute, set up a new NIH Planning Group on Clinical Trial Monitoring.

The British journal *The Lancet* called the whole affair "poorly handled," and editorialized that "The truth is that the overall trial results are unaffected (eg, concerning lumpectomy versus mastectomy) and that patients have no cause for concern on that count. The 'punishment' being meted out to Fisher by the NCI, by the National Institutes of Health, and by Congress...far and away exceeds the 'crime.'"[112]

By the summer of 1994 the National Cancer Institute had once again opened up ongoing trials to new participants, but the study of tamoxifen as a breast cancer preventative ran into heavy criticism.

RANDOMIZED CONTROLLED STUDIES

The tamoxifen (Breast Cancer Prevention Trial or BCPT) trial is a typical randomized controlled study, in which the participants must meet certain qualifications (such as additional risks for breast cancer) and are divided into two groups, one taking tamoxifen and the other a placebo, a harmless substance that looks like the actual medication.

In many of such studies neither the patient nor her doctor knows who is getting the real thing. This type of trial is known as a "double-blind" study; in a "single-blind," the patient doesn't know which group she is in, but doctors may.

Randomized, "double-blind" studies are considered the best of all trials, but critics argue that, in the case of tamoxifen, there is no need to expose healthy women to the possibility of uterine cancer. These are, however, healthy women "at risk," and the information that may result from this trial could be very important.

The authors of a clinical trial published in *The Lancet* advised that "...physicians should be alert to the higher risk of endometrial cancer in all women using tamoxifen, both breast cancer patients and healthy participants in prevention trials."[113]

PATIENTS AND CLINICAL TRIALS

In spite of their problems, clinical trials also offer participants many benefits, including being part of the latest treatments in the war against cancer. Cancer patients participating in a trial may sometimes experience a cure, or a longer time to live, and/or a better quality of life. There is always the chance, of course, that an experimental drug will hasten death or reduce the comfort and quality of life.

Many programs, especially those sponsored by the National Institutes of Health and the National Cancer Institute, are free to participants. And patients in such programs often receive medical care that is superior to standard treatment.

The way the plan is laid out for administration is called the Protocol. Often participants must follow a strict regimen, taking a precise amount of a drug, for instance, at precise times. They will also have certain tests administered at equally exact times.

If you enter a clinical trial, you may become part of a study testing one treatment on one group, or you may become part a study of one or more groups. One of the groups may receive "standard," or the most usual treatment, for the cancer. This is the "control" group. The "treatment" group or groups are the ones receiving the new drug or therapy.

If you wish to enter a particular trial, you may have to agree ahead of time to be "randomized"; that is, selected by chance (another roll of the dice!) for the control or the treatment group. No cancer patient, however, is placed in a control group with no treatment (such as a placebo) unless there is nothing known to be helpful in treating that particular cancer. Likewise, if the new treatment turns out to be harmful or too toxic, it will be stopped (or should be). If, on the other hand, the new treatment proves to be very effective, the trial is stopped and everyone receives the new therapy.

The Physician's Health Study, started in 1982 to compare the effectiveness of aspirin and beta carotene in 22,000 healthy male physicians, was "top drawer," or randomized, with half the participants taking 325 milligrams of aspirin every other day for 5 years and the other half taking a placebo. By 1988 it was obvious that aspirin was decreasing the risk of heart attacks in the treatment group, so everybody was given the chance to take aspirin.

Not every program proves that successful, of course, and a patient has the right to drop out of a trial at any time.

CLINICAL TRIAL PHASES

Clinical trials of new therapies are divided into phases, and cancer patients can participate in all of them.

Phase I. In this earliest phase, the new treatment is given to a small number of patients, usually people with advanced disease who are no longer benefiting from any treatment and are willing to take on the risks involved. Since the new treatment is highly experimental, those participating are taking a big gamble that the treatment will be more beneficial than toxic, but there is always the chance of a cure, or at least a longer life. Phase I trials basically start with the preliminaries -- to determine how patients react to the treatment and what the standard dosage should be.

Phase II. The treatment goes into Phase II only when Phase I has been successful. Now the treatment is tried on various types of cancer patients, generally those who have recurrent cancer but are not gravely ill. If some or all of the patients respond, then the program moves to Phase III.

Phase III. The new drug or other treatment is compared directly to a "standard" therapy to see which one is the more effective.

Phase IV. Because it has proved to be as good, or even better than a current or standard one, the new treatment becomes part of standard care itself. If it is a drug, it becomes part of the arsenal approved by the U.S. Food & Drug Administration for cancer therapy.

DRUG APPROVALS

On the average it takes 12 years and 231 million dollars to get a new drug on the market, according to the Pharmaceutical Manufacturers Association.

Only one in 4,000 compounds that start out in the lab make it to the market, according to the PMA, which claims that the U.S. system of new drug approval is probably the toughest in the world. All drugs for all medical purposes are supposed to go through the three-phase study process. Phase I lasts about a year, Phase II about two years, Phase III three years, and the Food and Drug Administration review process another two and a half. If the drug has shown sufficient promise against a serious or life-threatening illness such as cancer, Phases II and III can be combined to expedite the approval procedure.

GETTING INTO A CLINICAL TRIAL

In her book about the breast and breast cancer, Dr. Susan Love wrote, "Only about 3 percent of breast cancer patients in the United States participate in protocols [clinical trials]. This is much lower than in Europe and not something for us to be proud of."[114]

But clinical trials are available at research and hospital centers throughout the country. Your doctor may know of some in your area. If not, you can call the National Cancer Institute's Cancer Information Service at 1-800-4-CANCER for details. You can also use this number to order the NCI's brochure, *What Are Clinical Trials All About?* NCI also sponsors a treatment information system called PDQ which can give your doctor information on the latest trials being offered around the country for various stages of breast cancer.

The CCOP (Community Clinical Oncology Program) links community physicians with NCI clinical programs, allowing cancer patients to participate in trials within their own communities.

The National Institutes of Health, the parent organization of the NCI, runs many trials at its Bethesda, Maryland, facility just outside Washington, D.C. These studies are free to participants.

If you are eligible and want to enter a clinical trial, regardless of its location, you will go through a process called informed consent, which means you will be given information about the trial, the form or forms of treatment, and the possible risks as well as benefits. You'll have a chance to ask questions before deciding to participate in the program. If you decide to go ahead, you'll be given an informed consent form to read and consider before signing. You still have the right, however, to leave the program at any time.

Clinical trials do have protective features. Trials that are federally funded and regulated must first be approved by an Institutional Review Board, located at the place of the study. The IRB board, which includes scientists, doctors, lawyers, clergy and others from the community, reviews the study to make sure it is well designed and has patient safeguards as well as reasonable risks in relation to potential benefits.

Most trials are also subject to periodical reviews by researchers in other locations.

Although federal clinical trials, such as those at the National Institutes of Health, are free, others may not be. But you may be able to get financial aid through the social services office of the clinic or hospital sponsoring the trial. The Cancer Information Service (1-800-4-CANCER) and the American Cancer Society may also be able to give you sources for financial aid.

FLAWS

Since not everything in this world is perfect, clinical trials included, some studies can actually produce conflicting data.

One example of this confusion is caffeine. We've seen studies showing caffeine causes birth defects and even breast lumps. Other studies have exonerated caffeine. Researchers have also come up with varying results on the effects of alcohol on breast cancer risk and the value of antioxidants as cancer preventatives.

Some of these conclusions can come from faulty application of statistics, results that "are statistically significant...but aren't necessarily true," according to Rick Weiss in *The Washington Post Health* Magazine. "The lesson is not that statistics can't be trusted, but that numbers, like patients must be treated with care. In the words of one London epidemiologist: Just because a study shows that people who carry matches have a higher risk of lung cancer, don't assume that matches cause cancer."[115]

And then there is the business of mammograms for women aged 40 to 50. Some studies have indicated mammograms are inappropriate for this group, while others seemed to show that younger women should have *more* than older women!

One of the major problems with clinical trials may be ignorance, according to Richard Peto, clinical trialist with Oxford University, quoted in *Science*, the magazine of the American Association for the Advancement of Science. This situation is not surprising, according to *Science*, "...if one considers how much formal training in conducting clinical trials physicians receive: in many cases, none."[116]

In its special report on clinical trials, *Science* noted that "...NIH has no overall policy governing oversight of large, multi-site clinical trials. And since NIH currently sponsors more than 300 such trials, which shape health-care decisions for the entire country, the question of whether it should have an overall policy is a crucial one."[117]

Another problem with trials can result from media or medical overenthusiasm or social pressures. The Food and Drug Administration is subject to such pressures and can give permission for a drug to be used even before the long clinical process is completed, if the need is great. This is particularly true with drugs pertaining to AIDS and cancer.

One drug that may have been oversold is taxol, which was originally approved by the FDA for use in treatment-resistant ovarian cancer. Once on the market, however, a drug can be used by physicians as a treatment for anything, so breast cancer patients were receiving taxol treatment even before such use was approved. Although taxol has now been approved for advanced breast cancer, the drug has problems. It has been credited with striking remissions in some cancers, but the effects may be temporary and the toxicity is often terrible.

But in spite of their drawbacks, clinical trials are the backbone of the development and testing of new treatments for cancer and other diseases. While a careful review of drugs may occasionally delay a valuable drug's commercial use, the results and reviews of such trials may be our only assurance that the drugs we pay for, and submit to, are likely to be beneficial.

17. EPILOGUE
WHEN THE DICE FAIL:
ONE WOMAN'S STORY

I t started on an April morning several years ago. My husband and I had just returned from a European vacation, and I was about to call my friend Amy when she reached me.

"I've just had a mastectomy," Amy said.

Now, Amy was a warm, wonderful, witty friend of long standing, but she was also a hypochondriac, a terrible driver, and a bit of an hysteric. So her cheerful, matter-of-fact manner -- she might have been telling me she had just bought a new dress -- added to my shock.

And this was the first time breast cancer had struck a close friend. How could she be so damn calm?

And why a mastectomy? Amy and I were comfortable enough with each other -- we had been roommates, co-workers, and medical confidantes -- that I could ask.

The doctors had left the treatment choice up to her, Amy explained, and her fair, cancer-prone skin wasn't likely to tolerate radiation well.

Her underarm lymph nodes were clear, and there was no evidence of cancer spread, Amy told me, and no additional treatment was needed.

"So you had cancer but now you don't," I said with forced brightness, hoping I was right.

"That's what the doctor said, too," Amy agreed.

We were wrong.

I had never thought of Amy as especially courageous, and with her mercurial temperament and flair for hypochondria, she seemed a poor candidate for coping with a serious illness. I had a lot to learn about someone I had known for twenty-five years.

Amy was the first friend I made after college. She was already a fledgling reporter when I joined *The Washington Evening Star* as a typist/copy girl. While I sat at the reporters' table in the *Star's* cafeteria, listening in awed silence to repartee I was certain equaled any at the Algonquin Round Table, Amy actually participated in the conversation, and sometimes even *argued* with the older, established reporters.

Later I was one of Amy's roommates at her Georgetown apartment, a tiny two-bedroom affair that she somehow ended up sharing with three other young women. Things were so crowded that I slept on the living room couch. We didn't get much sleep, however, for our lives seemed in constant, albeit often pleasant, turmoil. Amy was the one who supplied the best, most level-headed advice about careers, love lives, and psyches, even though at the time she was undergoing her own psychological upheaval. (Once even left in an orphanage for a time, she had spent much of her childhood in strict boarding schools and was left intolerant of her own behavior and that of others. So she began the first of hundreds of therapeutic hours that turned her into an open-minded, open-hearted woman, wife, and mother.)

Amy had the smallest bedroom of the apartment to herself. She was then covering the *Star*'s evening diplomatic beat, and I awakened her every morning before I left for my own job, now in the editorial section of an insurance company. Amy looked so pretty in the morning. Her blond hair framed skin with a luminous rosiness, and her eyes would open big and hazy blue, surprised to see me there.

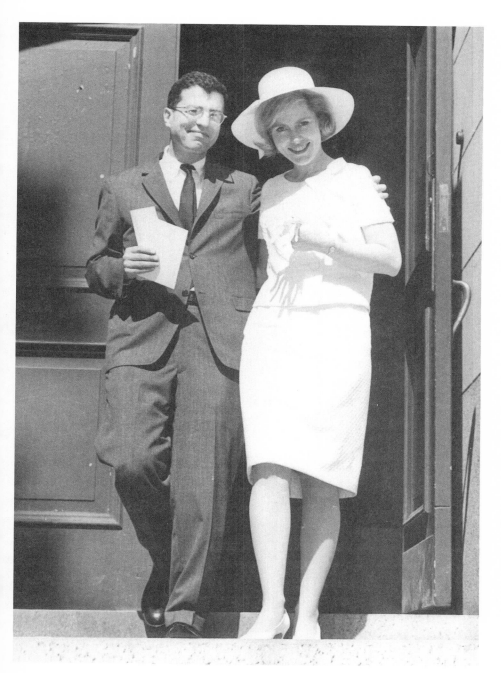

Amy and Irv Manning on their wedding day.

Three years later Amy became the first of us to marry. She remained a confidante, however, helping me and others, as she always had, through professional and romantic traumas.

Eventually she quit her job and became a full-time mother. When the children were two and five, Amy confessed one evening that she was suffering from cabin fever and wished she could find a local part-time job. I worked nearby and about that time my boss asked if I would like to share an additional employee with another division. Could we take on a part-time employee instead? I asked. So Amy came to work in my publications division. I was her boss -- supposedly.

The new relationship was not without its perils. Amy never paid attention to structured corporate behavior and would interrupt any meeting with an impervious "Martha!" when she wanted something. To the distress of our department head, who favored firmly structured office hours, Amy's working times fluctuated hourly. And neither she nor I could always control our tempers. On the other hand, in addition to her writing skills, she showed a flair for copy editing and a zany wit that soon enlivened our publications. She used the telephone as a fine-tuned instrument to elicit information, ignoring the secretarial chain of command to demand -- and get -- information from the company's top brass. She could reduce complex issues to understandable English and also showed a talent for teaching. Soon she was helping insurance technicians learn good written communications skills.

Before she left the company seven years later, Amy had recruited at least two friends as part-time employees, and their hours were just as complicated and fluctuating as hers had been.

When her girls entered their teens, Amy and her husband, Irv, moved from the Maryland suburbs just north of the District of Columbia to a house in Virginia not far from Mt. Vernon. The schools there seemed better, but Amy, a Washington native, was homesick. Although her intellect was at home almost everywhere, Amy didn't care for travel, and far-off Alexandria, Virginia, might just as well have been Los Angeles, California.

Amy was still in Alexandria when she went to the doctor to see about the breast lump she had found. But three months after the mastectomy she began to house-hunt in her old stomping grounds, and I tipped her off to a house coming up for sale directly behind my own. She was immediately on the phone to my brother-in-law, Bob, a real estate agent.

"I'll take it," she told him, even though she hadn't seen the inside of the place.

Amy had been with me the day Bob took me through my own house. "Buy it, buy it," Amy had whispered as we tromped through dark gray rooms. "You can always paint!"

Although Bob insisted Amy see the inside of the house before she purchased it, she was soon our back-door neighbor. I wasn't the only one thrilled to have her back "in town," and one friend threw a big "welcome back" dinner party.

Amy had a knack for decorating, and her new house soon reflected her talent. Although her style was consistent, nothing in the house was cast in stone -- moving furniture was a form of therapy as well as one of her few forms of exercise. Her flair for decorating extended to advising her friends. "The desk has to be under the window," she told me when I consulted her about creating a bedroom office area. Within minutes she was rearranging the furniture.

In addition to an enviable collection of Oriental carpets, Amy crocheted her own rugs and even made some for close friends. I have mine near my desk under the window.

So Amy was back in town and, for two years after her operation, she was fine, just coping with the usual problems: Too little time, a hectic editing and writing job with McGraw-Hill, pretty daughters about to enter adulthood. Then, abruptly, she was hospitalized with a mysterious fluid buildup in her heart and liver. After a number of appalling tests, she called me from the hospital.

"They've found breast cancer cells in the fluid," she said, her voice almost a whisper. The cancer had spread to the pericardial sac that surrounds the heart.

Amy planned her job schedule around the chemotherapy injections that followed, staying home the first days after the treatment, then gradually lengthening her workweek until it was time for another shot. She hated the chemotherapy and one day, just a few months later, called to announce she was going off it for good. "I feel better already," she said, her voice ebullient.

I wasn't quite so sure. I never did understand why the doctors allowed her to go off the chemotherapy so soon.

There were ups and downs for the next months, and then the cancer struck again. New chemotherapy was prescribed. It made her lose some hair, but Amy bought a flattering wig that looked real and declared her immune system ready for a fight.

Her friends were part of that fight. She had a particular knack for sharing, somehow penetrating our shields of privacy. Willingly, we learned cancer's course just as we had shared with Amy our concerns about our homes, husbands, careers, children. Most people count close friends on the fingers of one hand; with Amy it took piano keys. College classmates, former roommates, former and current neighbors, workmates, members of a book club, a therapy group (therapy had become one of Amy's hobbies), all were part of her entourage.

Because of her candor, we friends lived with the cancer, too, participating in the one-step-forward, two-steps-back progress of her disease. We felt the anger generated by a sometimes unfeeling or incompetent physician. We wondered at the calm and courage of this self-confessed hypochondriac who had once complained of pregnancy and premature menopause within a single week. We marveled as death's approach strengthened and ennobled Amy's already loving relationship with her husband, Irv.

Even before the next horror -- a brain tumor -- we were already telling one another that Amy was setting the standard for the rest of us.

Amy gloried in a brief euphoria produced by a steroid treatment for her brain tumor. "What a marvelous gift this has been," she told me several times during the Christmas holidays in that whispery voice we both knew probably came from some unidentified metastasis.

In January I told Amy about a dream I'd had. It was set at a local hospital, where Amy had been visiting a doctor. When I arrived to meet her there, she had left a message for me to call her. I was to borrow her doctor's plane and fly over to meet her at a nearby airport. "It's just around the corner," she explained over the phone. "Once you're here, I'll take over."

I had a terrible time finding the doctor -- the offices were all deserted except for one with a bag man in it. Eventually, however, I located the doctor, who stopped moving only long enough to tell me that, yes, I could borrow his plane.

I was terrified but went to the airport -- right next to the hospital in the dream -- partly because Amy was again on the telephone giving me instructions. Pretty soon some technicians were rolling out the plane, which looked old and decrepit. But there was Amy on the phone again, calling me from *her* airport, just down the road. "Don't worry," she said. "All you have to do is get to me and I'll do the rest. I'll teach you to fly."

By this time the sun was starting to sink, and soft streaks of white, blue, and pink clouds were painted across the deep blue sky. As I stood, shaking, Amy kept saying, "There's nothing to it. Just fly to me and then I'll show you how easy it is."

I was scared stiff. The lights of the city began to come on, the planes in silhouette now. But as the blues and pinks in the sky grew more brilliant against the darkening sky, I was drawn to the doctor's plane. I entered it just as the sun started to sink behind the horizon in a shower of gold. And Amy was saying, "Don't be afraid to fly, Martha. Just get to where I am and I will get you home. I will teach you to fly."

Amy and I both thought this was a pretty remarkable dream since she didn't like to travel *or* fly.

Later that month the steroids caused an embolism in her lung, and Amy, facing a life-threatening procedure, called me from the hospital. She had already had a pre-operative shot, she told me in a whispery voice, but she wanted me to know that she had already planned the kind of ceremony she wanted after her death.

"Oh, Amy!" I protested. The word death hadn't been mentioned aloud before.

I cried silently, as Amy explained: "I want the ceremony at home. It won't be terribly religious, although there will be Bible readings." Tom, a friend and non-practicing priest, would be "master of ceremonies, so to speak." There would be favorite poetry and music, remarks by the immediate family. "I've asked some friends to read, some from their own works. And I'd like you to tell about the flying dream you had," Amy said. "I like the symbolism."

She lived through the embolism crisis and there was a brief respite, although she was now taking pain killers regularly. Amazingly, she remained responsive to the needs of those around her. She wept with me when our dog died, saying that bereavement leave should extend to pets. I gave her the opening chapters of a mystery novel I was writing. It was set on a ship. "I can't seem to get into the story," she said apologetically sometime later, "but it's probably my illness." I read the chapters over and discovered that the problem had nothing to do with Amy's cancer; the problem had to do with me. The writing dragged like a grounded boat.

I started over.

As spring came, Amy's doctor told her she was holding her own and didn't have to see him again until June. "I didn't think I'd *be* here in June," she told me, amazement in her voice.

A few days later she was calling me about a new breast lump. It, too, was malignant, but this time there was no mastectomy. Amy's lungs weren't in good enough shape for anything but local anesthesia.

Not long afterwards I came over for tea. Amy was up and around, pretty in a loose pink outfit. She certainly didn't look like someone with serious cancer. I told her so. She agreed, then described the latest findings, the latest medicines. "Oh, Martha!" she said, fear in those blue-gray eyes.

Perhaps it was because I was unaccepting or simply because she looked so good that we didn't talk about the cancer anymore that day. Amy promised to come to a big party my husband, Bill, and I were having in early May -- so many mutual friends would be there. But she wouldn't stay long. "I don't have much endurance," she explained apologetically.

The morning of the party she called. "The irises are in full bloom by the garage door," she said. "They are so pretty. Please take as many as you can use for decoration."

I thanked her and said I'd see her later.

But Amy didn't come to the party. Just as the last guests were leaving, Irv called. Amy had had trouble breathing, he said, and he had taken her to the emergency room. She was soon home again, on new medicine, but it was obvious that cancer had invaded her lungs. Oxygen was added to her treatments.

A couple of weeks later Irv invited me over for a drink. Amy's sister, Mary, was in town, he said, and Amy wanted me to meet her.

At first Mary's ebullience was almost enough to cover the obvious decline I saw in Amy's condition. She was seated in the living room, an invalid now, her voice only a husky gasp.

I learned almost between the lines what an effort it had been for her to make an appearance.

Mary and I made bright small talk while occasionally Amy struggled to speak, telling me that a hospice nurse was to start coming in.

During the next few weeks Amy or Irv would call occasionally, asking for a small favor of some sort. Bill and I were grateful for any chance to help -- it was frustrating being close neighbors and friends with little to do.

One day I asked Any if she would like anything special to eat. No, she replied. Nothing tasted good.

"Custard?" I had made it for her before.

"Well, custard. But, oh, it's so much trouble," she whispered.

I made the custard the next day and passed it over the fence.

The following Saturday Irv brought a note from Amy. Underneath Mary Cassatt's painting of a sulky "Child in a Straw Hat," Amy had written, "This little girl did not get any of Martha Grigg's custard. What she is thinking is not 'Oh, shucks.'"

I was very touched by the note and even more, pleasurably surprised to see an example of Amy's humor, written in a strong hand. Her physical state, particularly her voice, seemed so weak that subconsciously, I suppose, I had assumed her mind was similarly affected.

Irv mentioned something about taking Amy out for a ride in the wheelchair, and I was surprised. I hadn't known about the wheelchair.

Bill and I went to a dance that night and brought home the flowers from our table. It was a hot, beautiful June morning when we passed them over the fence for Amy. "She has really enjoyed the custard," Amy's daughter said.

That night Irv called to say that Amy might not live until morning. Did I want to say goodbye?

I fought tears as I entered the bedroom. Amy's eyes were closed. There was an oxygen tube in her nose. Baby-like wisps of hair framed her face.

"Martha is here, darling," Irv said gently.

Amy's eyes opened in surprise. They were the same big blue eyes in the flushed pretty face I remembered from a Georgetown apartment a generation ago. Amy tried to speak, but Irv had told me she no longer could. I sat beside the bed, holding her hand, as Amy, her half-closed eyes shaded by long black lashes, went in and out of consciousness.

I babbled on, telling her how much I would and did miss her. Who would tell me where to put the furniture? How to revise a story? Cope with a husband in mid-life crisis?

Remus, Amy's Belgian sheep dog, came up silently, wanting to be petted. I stroked the long black fur, wondering if his sad eyes reflected some inner knowledge.

I glanced around the room, at the soft pink and blue sheets on the bed, the unobtrusive oxygen container. The gallant way Amy and Irv, too, had lived through her illness seemed to come together in this room -- the soft light, the articles of the gravely ill clustered but not cluttered near the bed. This was a sick room somehow enveloped in love and dignity, with the big old dog still welcome, loving daughters and husband only a room away. If you had to die, this was the place to do it. And that fit the pattern. For Amy had brought us along step-by-step, setting the standard.

I remembered the flying dream, of Amy saying, "I will get you home. I will teach you to fly."

She had taught us all.

NOTES

1. NIH Congressional Luncheon Series, Oct 5, 1992

2. Brochure: Research on Breast Cancer/Pharmaceutical Manufacturers Assoc., 1993

3. Early Breast Trialists' Collaborative Group, "Systemic Treatment of early breast cancer by hormonal, cytotoxic, or immune therapy," *The Lancet*, Jan 4 & 11, 1992

4. Andrew A. Skolnick, "New Data Suggest Needle Biopsies Could Replace Surgical Biopsy for Diagnosing Breast Cancer," pp. 1724-28, *Journal of the American Medical Association (JAMA)*, 6/8/94.

5. William L. Donegan, M.D., "Evaluation of A Palpable Breast Mass," p. 937, *The New England Journal of Medicine*, 9/24/92

6. Reported by *The New York Times* & American Cancer Society, 5/25/94

7. Samuel Broder at a National Cancer Advisory Board Meeting, 1/10/95

8. At a My Image Open Door Program, 11/14/92, Bethesda, MD

9. Joseph P. Crowe, Jr., et al., "Age Does Not Predict Breast Cancer Outcomes," *Archives of Surgery*, pp. 483-88, May 1994

10. At an NIH Press Conference, 9/14/94

11. Martha L. Slattery, PhD., & Richard A. Kerber, PhD., "A Comprehensive Evaluation of Family History...," pp. 1563-68, and Barbara L. Weber, M.D., and Judy E. Garber, M.D., editorial, pp. 1602-3, *JAMA*, 10/6/93

12. "Add Another Risk Factor," p. 2, *Images, Newsletter of My Image After Breast Cancer*, November 1993

13. As reported in *Internal Medicine News & Cardiology News*, p.29, 9/15/92

14. Ron Winslow, "Study Finds Pill Poses Little Risk of Breast Cancer," Wall Street Journal, p. B-7, 4/6/94

15. Graham A. Colditz, M.B., B.S., et al., "The Use of Estrogens and Progestins and the Risk of Breast Cancer in Postmenopausal Women," pp 1589-93, *The New England Journal of Medicine*, 6/15/95

16. Bruce Jancin, "How Estrogen Therapy Cuts CHD Mortality," p. 43, *Internal Medicine News & Cardiology News*, 4/15/94

17. Associated Press report in *The Washington Post*, 5/18/94

18. Erik L. Goldman, "Even 'Social Drinking' May Raise Lifetime Risk of Breast Cancer," *Family Practice News*, p. 12, 12/1/93

19. Peter Gorner, "Statistics Give Confusing, Alarming View," *Chicago Tribune*, 4/10/94

20. Nancy Krieger et al.,"Breast Cancer and Serum Organochlorines: Prospective Study Among White, Black and Asian Women," p. 589, *Journal of the National Cancer Institute (NCI)*, 4/20/94

21. Anders Mattsson et al. "Radiation-Induced Breast Cancer: Long-Term Follow-up of Radiation Therapy for Benign Breast Disease," p. 1679, *Journal of the NCI*, 10/20/93

22. Susan Jenks, "News," p. 578, *Journal of the NCI*, 4/20/94

23. "News," p. 1629, *Journal of the NCI*, 10/20/93

24. Rick Weiss, "Linking Physical and Emotional Health," p. 8, *The Washington Post Health Magazine*, 1/11/94

25. Bernard Fisher, et al., "Endometrial Cancer in Tamoxifen-Treated Breast Cancer Patients"...(Project NSABP, B-14), pp. 527-37, *Journal of the NCI*, 4/6/94

26. Flora E van Leeuwen et al., "Risk of Endometrial Cancer after Tamoxifen Treatment of Breast Cancer," pp. 448f, *The Lancet*, 2/19/94

27. Gladys Block, editorial, pp. 846-8, *Journal of the NCI*, 6/2/93

28. Reported in *The New York Times* & others, 4/12/94

29. Fawn Vrazo, "Study: Breast Milk Reduces Cancer Risk," p. A-3, *Philadelphia Inquirer*, 5/2/94

30. K. Smigel, "Dietary Supplements Reduce Cancer Deaths in China," p. 1448, *Journal of the NCI*, 9/15/93

31. "Sorting Out the Beta Carotene Study," Jane E. Brody, Personal Health Column, p. C-11, *The New York Times*, 4/20/94

32. Meera Jain et al., "Premorbid Diet and the Prognosis of Women with Breast Cancer," pp 1390-97, *Journal of the NCI*, 9/21/94

33. Leslie Bernstein et al., "Physical Exercise and Reduced Risk of Breast Cancer in Young Women," pp. 1403-8, *Journal of the NCI*, 9/21/94

34. Jane E. Brody, [Mammograms under age 50] "Some Radiologists Say Benefit Exists and Will Emerge in Time," p. C-1, *The New York Times*, 12/14/93

35. Malcolm Gladwell, "How Safe Are Your Breasts?" pp.22f, *The New Republic*, 10/24/94

36. Hyman B. Muss, M.D., "c-erbB-2 Expression and Response to Adjuvant Therapy in Women with Node-Positive Early Breast Cancer," p. 1260f, and Aron Goldhirse, M.D. & Richard D. Gelber, PhD., "Understanding Adjuvant Chemotherapy for Breast Cancer," p. l308f, *The New England Journal of Medicine*, 5/5/94,

37. Robert Berkow, M.D., editor-in-chief, p. 1818, *The Merck Manual*, 16th edition, Merck Research Labs, 1992

38. "Microvessels in Breast DCIS," p. 571, (Guidi et al., pp.614f), *Journal of the NCI*, 4/20/94

39. *Dr. Susan Love's Breast Book* with Karen Lindsey, Addison-Wesley Publishing Co., 1990 & 91, p. 270

40. Joyce Wadler, *My Breast*, p. 34, Addison-Wesley Pub. Co., 1992

41. Bernard Fisher, M.D., et al., "Lumpectomy Compared with Lumpectomy and Radiation Therapy for the Treatment of Intraductal Breast Cancer," pp. 1581-6, *The New England Journal of Medicine*, 6/3/93

42. My Image Open Door Program, Bethesda, MD., 11/14/92

43. Anna Lee-Feldstein, PhD, et al., "Treatment Differences and Other Prognostic Factors Related to Breast Cancer Survival," pp. 1163-68, *JAMA*, 4/20/94

44. Arthur E. Baue, M.D., "Breast Conservation Operations for Treatment of Cancer of the Breast," pp. 1204-5, *JAMA*, 4/20/94

45. At a National Cancer Institute Workshop: "An Appraisal of Clinical Research for the Treatment of Early Breast Cancer," Bethesda, MD, 11/15/94

46. John&LeeZa TV show, Oct. 25, 1993

47. Jay Siwek, M.D., "Quitting Smoking before Surgery," p. 15, *The Washington Post Health* Magazine, 9/22/92

48. Umberto Veronesi, M.D., et al., "Effect of Menstrual Phase on Surgical Treatment of breast cancer," pp. 1544-46, *The Lancet*, 6/18/94

49. Frank Field, "A Simple Treatment Convinces the Skeptics," p. 20, *Parade Magazine*, 9/4/94

50. Donald J. Ferguson, "Questions and Answers," p. 503, *JAMA*, 2/8/95

51. Bernard J. Colan, "Surgeons and Patients Need Education on Benefit of PT following Mastectomy and Breast Reconstruction," p. 4, *ADVANCE for Physical Therapists* newsletter, 4/4/94

52. Umberto Veronesi, M.D. et al., "Radiotherapy after Breast-Preserving Surgery in Women with Localized Cancer of the Breast," p. 1589, *The New England Journal of Medicine*, 6/3/94

53. NCI Workshop, "An Appraisal of Clinical Research for the Treatment of Early Breast Cancer," Bethesda. MD, 11/15/94

54. Ibid

55. Early Breast Cancer Trialists' Collaborative Group, "Systemic Treatment of Early Breast Cancer by Hormonal, Cytotoxic or Immune Therapy," and discussion, *The Lancet*, 1/11/92

56. William C. Wood, M.D., et al., "Dose and Dose Intensity of Adjuvant Chemotherapy for Stage II, Node-positive Breast Carcinoma," p. 1253f, *The New England Journal of Medicine*, 5/5/94

57. Gina Kolata, "Study Backs Chemotherapy Regimen," *The New York Times*, 5/5/94

58. Aron Goldhirsch, M.D. & Richard D. Gelber, PhD., "Understanding Adjuvant Chemotherapy for Breast Cancer," p. 1308, *The New England Journal of Medicine*, 5/5/94

59. Hyman B. Muss, M.D., "c-*erb*B-2 Expression and Response to Adjuvant Therapy in Women with Node-Positive Early Breast Cancer," p. 1260f, *The New England Journal of Medicine*, 5/5/94

60. William C. Wood, M.D., et al., "Dose and Dose Intensity of Adjuvant Chemotherapy for Stage II, Node-Positive Breast Carcinoma," p. 1259, *The New England Journal of Medicine*, 5/5/94

61. William Hrushesky, M.D., "Diminishing Breast Cancer Chemotherapy by Respecting Biological Rhythms," *Y-ME Hotline Newsletter*, Sept/Oct & Nov/Dec 1993

62. Yashar Hirshaut & Peter I. Pressman, *Breast Cancer/The Complete Guide*, pp. 176 & 177, Bantam Books, 1992

63. Early Breast Cancer Trialists' Collaborative Group, "Systemic Treatment of Early Breast Cancer by Hormonal, Cytotoxic, or Immune Therapy," and editorials, *The Lancet*, 1/4/92 & 1/11/92

64. Richard Gray, Editorial: "Tamoxifen: How Boldly to Go Where No Women have Gone Before," p. 1358, *Journal of the NCI*, 9/1/93

65. Lisa Seachrist, "Tamoxifen: Hanging in the Balance," p. 1525, *Science*, 6/10/94

66. NCI Press Release, 3/29/94

67. Eliot Marshall, Ibid, *Science*, p. 1525

68. FDA Press Release, 4/7/94

69. NCI Press Release, 5/16/94

70. Linda Carroll, "Tamoxifen's Suggested Link to Endometrial Cancer in Doubt," *Medical Tribune*, 3/10/94

71. Rajendra P. Kedar et al, "Effects of Tamoxifen on Uterus and Ovaries of Postmenopausal Women in a Randomised Breast Cancer Prevention Trial," p. 1318, *The Lancet*, 5/28/94

72. NCI Workshop, "An Appraisal of Clinical Research for the Treatment of Early Breast Cancer," 11/15/94

73. "Adjuvant Tamoxifen Therapy for Early Stage Breast Cancer and Second Primary Malignancies," Lars E. Rutqvist et al., *Journal of the NCI*, pp 645-651, 5/3/95

74. NCI/NSABP Press Release, 4/29/92

75. NCI Press Release, 5/2/95

76. Richard R. Love, M.D., et al.,"Effects of Tamoxifen on Bone Mineral Density in Postmenopausal Women with Breast Cancer," pp. 853f, *The New England Journal of Medicine*, 3/26/94

77. Peter Martin, "From Darkness Into Light," *The London Sunday Times Magazine*, 4/11/93

78. Editorial: "Ovarian Ablation in Early Breast Cancer: Phoenix Arisen?" p. 95, 1/11/92, *The Lancet*

79. Ibid, *The London Sunday Times Magazine*, 4/11/93

80. NCI Workshop, "An Appraisal of Clinical Research for the Treatment of Early Breast Cancer," 11/15/94

81. "Health Hotline," p. 13, *Bottom Line/Personal*, 8/15/92

82. "Foreword," Robert Berkow, M.D., Editor-in-Chief, *The Merck Manual, Sixteenth Edition*, Merck Research Laboratories, 1992

83. Lisa M. Orange, "Breast Cancer Evokes Serious Psychiatric Reaction in 20% of Patients," p. 7, *Family Practice News*, 7/1/93

84. Katherine A. Billingham, PhD, *Y-ME Hotline Newsletter*, Jan/Feb 1993

85. Peter Martin, "From Darkness into Light," *The London Sunday Times Magazine*, 4/11/93

86. Elisabeth Rosenthal, "Listening to the Emotional Needs of Cancer Patients," p. C-1, *The New York Times*, 7/22/93

87. Abigail Van Buren, "Mastectomy Isn't the End of the World," p. B-5, "Dear Abby," *The Washington Times*, 9/15/92

88. Marion Morra and Eve Potts, *CHOICES: Realistic Alternatives in Cancer Treatment*, p. 362, Avon Books, 1980 & 87

89. Rachel Urquhart, "Great Hair!" p. 168, *Vogue Magazine*, July 1992

90. D. V. Schapira & Nicole Urban, "A Minimalist Policy for Breast Cancer Surveillance," p. 380, *JAMA*, 1/16/91

91. Marco Rosselli Del Turco, M.D., et al., "Intensive Diagnostic Follow-up after Treatment of Primary Breast Cancer," p. 1596, *JAMA*, 5/25/94

92. My Image Open Door Meeting, March 1992

93. Samuel Broder, Address to National Cancer Advisory Board, 1/10/95

94. Corinna Nelson, "News," *Journal of the NCI*, pp 1753-54, 1/5/94

95. "Ask the Doctor," by Colleen Hagen, M.D., *Y-ME Hotline Newsletter*, Sept/Oct 1992

96. Romano Demicheli et al.,"Local Recurrences Following Mastectomy: Support for the Concept of Tumor Dormancy," pp. 45-46, *Journal of the NCI*, 1/5/94

97. *Breast Cancer/The Complete Guide*, by Yashar Hirshaut and Peter I. Pressman, Bantam Books, 1992, p. 236

98. Hyman B. Muss, M.D., "Interrupted Versus Continuous Chemotherapy in Patients with Metastatic Breast Cancer," p. 1344, *The New England Journal of Medicine*, 11/7/91

99. Kathy Christman, M.D., et al., The Piedmont Oncoloy Assoc. Experience, "Chemotherapy of Metastatic Breast Cancer in the Elderly," pp. 57-62, *JAMA*, 7/1/92

100.Peter Martin, "From Darkness into Light, *The London Sunday Times Magazine*, 4/11/93

101. *The Wall Street Journal*, 3/29/93

102. "The Blue Sheet," F.D.C. Reports, Inc., p. 6, 9/1/93

103. Andrea Martoni, et al., "Correspondence" -- "Antihistamines in the Treatment of Taxol-Induced Paroxystic Pain Syndrome," p. 676, *Journal of the NCI*, 4/21/93

104. William Boly, "Wishing on a Falling Star," pp. 63-69, *Health* Magazine, Sept. 1993

105. Charles L. Vogel, M.D., "Navelbine: The Forgotten Investigational New Drug," *Y-ME Hotline Newsletter*, Jan/Feb 1994

106. FDA Oncology Drugs Advisory Committee meeting, 6/7/94

107. Reported in *The Washington Post* and *The New York Times*, 4/12/94

108. Susan Jenks, "News," *Journal of the NCI*, p. 1629, 10/20/93

109. Calvin Price, "Pain Control Woefully Inadequate for....Many Patients," *Family Practice News*, 3/15/93

110. Cancer Pain Management Press Conference, March 2, 1994, Washington, D.C.

111. Frederick P. Smith, M.D., "Pain Management," *The Washington Clinic Newsletter*, Sept, 1992

112. Editorial: "Breast Cancer: Clearing Trails in the Forest without Losing Our Way," p. 1049, *The Lancet*, 4/30/94

113. Flora E van Leeuwen et al., "Risk of Endometrial Cancer after Tamoxifen Treatment of Breast Cancer," p. 451, *The Lancet*, 2/19/94

114. *Dr. Susan Love's Breast Book*, with Karen Lindsey, p. 216, Addison Wesley Publishing Co., 1990 & 1991

115. Rick Weiss, "Dazzled by Tortured Data," p. 6, *The Washington Post Health* Magazine, 11/23/93

116. Rachel Nowak, "Ignorance Is Not Bliss: A Close Look at Clinical Trials," p. 1538, *Science*, 6/10/94

117. Rachel Nowak, "Clinical Trial Monitoring: Hit or Miss? A Close Look at Clinical Trials," p. 1534, *Science*, 6/10/94

INDEX